T0133336

THE WONDERFUL ART OF THE EYE

Medieval Texts and Studies
General Editor: John A. Alford

Benvenutus Grassus

The Wonderful Art of the Eye

A Critical Edition of the Middle English Translation
of his *De Probatissima Arte Oculorum*

Edited by L. M. Eldredge

Michigan State University Press
East Lansing

All Michigan State University Press books are produced on paper which meets the requirements of American National Standard of Information Sciences—Permanence of paper for printed materials ANSI Z39.48-1984.

Michigan State University Press
East Lansing, Michigan 48823-5202

03 02 01 00 99 98 97 96 1 2 3 4 5 6 7 8 9

ISBN 0-87013-459-0

A Colleagues Book

For Karin

CONTENTS

ACKNOWLEDGEMENTS

I should like to record here my gratitude to all the libraries in which I consulted manuscripts, read books, consulted librarians, and generally made a nuisance of myself. There is no more congenial environment for reading, writing, and contemplation than the libraries I have frequented, and I am grateful to them all for putting their resources at my disposal. Specifically, I should like to thank the librarian, Glasgow University Library, for his kind permission to quote from two manuscripts, Hunter V.8.6 (503) and Hunter V.8.16 (513). And I should like also to record my gratitude to the Bodleian Library, Oxford, for permission to quote from their manuscript Ashmole 1468, and to the British Library, London, for permission to quote from their manuscript Sloane 661.

I am also extremely grateful to the Hannah Institute for the History of Medicine, Toronto, for their continued support of this project. They provided the initial grant for the purchase of microfilms, both Latin and English, on which this edition and an earlier article are based, and they also provided a generous subvention to help pay the publication costs of this book.

Personally, my debts are many, and the few thanks I can give here are scant recompense to scholars whose courteous attempts to answer my queries and provide help have been unfailing. In order to avoid a massive list, I shall mention only those who have contributed directly to the preparation of this edition, but others to whom my debts are more general will, I hope, realize that they too are included in this expression of gratitude. As well as providing invaluable assistance at various stages along the way, Linda Ersam Voigts first drew my attention to MS Hunter V.8.16. Emilie Savage-Smith was most helpful in introducing me to Arabic ophthalmology, and I am also grateful to her for reading through an earlier paper on Benvenutus, as well as hearing me out on other ophthalmological matters. Inez Violé O'Neill made some fruitful suggestions in connection with the dating of Benvenutus, and Mr. V. J. Marmion, FRCSEd., FRCPE, was kind enough to comment on an earlier draft of this edition. I am especially grateful to the series editor, John A. Alford, for his patience, cooperation, and suggestions. And despite my relying so heavily on their sound advice, errors that may remain are my sole responsibility.

Ottawa and Oxford
Spring 1995

ABBREVIATIONS

adj.   adjective

adv.   adverb

CL   Classical Latin

conj.   conjunction

cp.   compare

DNB   George Smith, Leslie Stephen, Sidney Lee, et al.,
            eds., *Dictionary of National Biography*, 21 vols. plus
            supplements (London: Oxford University Press,
            1917–)

EETS OS   Early English Text Society, Original Series

Eng   English

fr   from

Gr   Greek

Hunt   Tony Hunt, *Plant Names of Medieval England*
            (Cambridge: Brewer, 1989)

indef.   indefinite

L   Latin

lit.   literal(ly)

ME   Middle English

MED	Hans Kurath, Sherman M. Kuhn, Robert E. Lewis, eds., *MiddleEnglish Dictionary* (Ann Arbor: University of Michigan Press, 1956–), complete through *tastinge* when this edition completed
ML	Medieval Latin
MLD	R. E. Latham and D. R. Howlett, eds., *Dictionary of Medieval Latin from British Sources* (London: British Academy, 1975–), complete through H when this edition completed
MS(S)	manuscript(s)
n.	noun
OE	Old English
NE	Modern English
OED	J. A. Simpson and E. S. C. Weiner, eds., *The Oxford English Dictionary*, 2nd ed. (Oxford: Clarendon, 1989)
ON	Old Norse
pl.	plural
p(p).	page(s)
pp.	past participle
prep.	preposition
pres.	present tense
pron.	pronoun
sing.	singular

T and K	Lynn Thorndike and Pearl Kibre, *A Catalogue of Incipits of Medieval Scientific Writings in Latin* (Cambridge, Mass.: Mediaeval Academy of America, 1963)
var.	variant
v.	verb

Latin Manuscripts Cited

Am	Erfurt, Wissenschaftliche Bibliothek, MS Amplonianische Q.193
P	Forlì, Biblioteca Communale Aurelio Saffi, collezioni Piancastelli, Sala O, MSS 111/49
N	Naples, Biblioteca Nazionale, MS VIII.G.100
VP1	Vatican, Biblioteca Apostolica, MS Palat. Lat. 1254
VP2	Vatican, Biblioteca Apostolica, MS Palat. Lat. 1268
VP3	Vatican, Biblioteca Apostolica, MS Palat. Lat. 1320
VR	Vatican, Biblioteca Apostolica, MS Regin. Lat. 373
VV	Vatican, Biblioteca Apostolica, MS Vat. Lat. 5373

Biography

THE EXISTENCE OF Benvenutus Grassus is attested only by his treatise on eye diseases and injuries. His name appears on no list of university lecturers, no manorial or monastic account book, no chronicle, no treatise on another subject. In short we have no details of his life except those that can be inferred from his work on ophthalmology. Even his name is subject to variation, many manuscripts calling him Grapheus or Graffeus, one even calling him Craston, and the French translation thinks of him as Raffe. Even Benvenutus comes in for its share of variety, ranging from Benvengut in Provençal and Bienvenu in French to curious spellings of the Latin.

Most scholars today agree to call him Benvenutus Grassus. Most also agree that he was in all probability a Christian and an Italian — the surname Grasso is still common in southern Italy — perhaps he was even a Neapolitan.[1] Various details in his treatise suggest that he travelled fairly widely — throughout Italy certainly, probably into North Africa among Berber tribes, perhaps too into France. The evidence for his excursions is the place-names he mentions in dealing with specific dis-

---

[1] The most extensive biography of Benvenutus is that of Noè Scalinci, "Questioni biografiche su Benvenuto Grasso jerosolimitano," *Atti e Memorie dell'Accademia di Storia dell'Arte Sanitaria*, ser. 2, 1 (1935), 190–205, 240–255, and 299–313. Scalinci should be read with some caution, however. He lacks any sense of scepticism about manuscripts and early printed editions and often accepts as definitive a reading that appears only in a single late manuscript. He is also concerned to show that Arabic medicine had no influence on Benvenutus and that all his learning could have been derived from Celsus and other Romans. Finally, he was himself a Neapolitan and perhaps wanted to claim Benvenutus as one of his early fellow townsmen. Scalinci's notes include references to all earlier studies of Benvenutus's biography.

eases and injuries, and these names divide into two types. One is the sort of remark that often comes at the end of an account of a disease, where he will say in what town or province he found this disease most prevalent. For example, he mentions Tuscany and the Marches as the places where the second type of phlegmatic disease is most prevalent, the third he found most in Sardinia, and the fourth among the Berbers in North Africa. He speaks of curing a boy's injured eye in Messina and of removing the beard of an ear of grain from the eye of a man in Lucca. The second type of place name comes when Benvenutus supplies a list of synonyms for a disease or a herb. For example, when he mentions a herb that he calls the most holy herb *candela saracenica* (*sanctissima herba quam uocamus candelam saracenicam* [N, f. 62v]), he goes on to note that the Arabs call it *tufefam*, the Greeks call it *sucum*, the Apulians call it *carducellum benedictum*, the Salernitans *lactucellam*, the Romans *crispinum*, and others from unspecified places call it *cressionum*. In dealing with a sty, he tells us that the Tuscans call it *humor benedictus*, the Romans *nexionam*, Sicilians and Greeks *papula*, and northern people and the French call it *humor maledictus*.

Of these two types of place names, one in connection with places where he has observed certain illnesses or treated certain injuries and the other in connection with a list of synonyms, it seems to me that we can put a fair amount of trust in the former and less in the latter. The synonyms serve two purposes: they extend the usefulness of the treatise by providing vocabulary for physicians that they can use in various places, and at the same time they make the author look more learned and experienced. But they are clearly names he could have gathered from texts or from conversations with travellers without ever having been near the places mentioned. But I have to believe him when he tells me of an incident in Lucca or Messina or that he found a certain disease more prevalent in one place than in another.

Establishing when he lived is more difficult. The earliest manuscript is probably that of the Provençal translation: Basel, Öffentliche Bibliothek der Universität, MS D.II.11, ff. 172–177v. This translation, which breaks off after the phlegmatic diseases, has been dated thirteenth century,[2] and so Benvenutus must have lived and written some time earlier than or contemporary with the date of the manuscript. To be sure a hundred years is a long time, but I think some evidence suggests that he lived rather later than earlier in the century. The first bit of evidence is the word *anatomy*, or *anothomie*, that recurs throughout this translation and in all the Latin manuscripts. The origin of this word is the Greek ανατομη, which means dissection, but in medieval medicine up to the thirteenth century the term *anatomia* usually means no more than a systematic knowledge of the human body, knowledge usually acquired from authorities.[3] In the thirteenth century, probably more gradually than suddenly, the practice of dissection resumed.[4] One group of Latin manuscripts, a group attesting to a somewhat later version than the English translation, carries a revised anatomical section which seems to

[2]The date, thirteenth to fourteenth century, is reported in A. M. Berger and T. M. Auracher, *Des Benvenutus Grapheus "Practica oculorum": Beitrag zur Geschichte der Augenheilkunde* (Munich, 1884), 13. They rely on Wilhelm Wackernagel, "Provenzalische Diätetik," *Zeitschrift für deutsches Altertum* 5 (1845), 16–17, whose brief opinion ("von einer [Hand] des 13n oder 14n . . .") has never, to my knowledge, been challenged.

[3]The early history of dissection can be found in Ludwig Edelstein, "Die Geschichte der Sektion in der Antike," *Quellen und Studien zur Geschichte der Naturwissenschaften und der Medizin*, Band 3, Heft 2 (Berlin: Julius Springer, 1932), 50–106 (continuous pagination pp. 100–156); translated in Oswei Temkin and C. Lillian Temkin, *Ancient Medicine: Selected Papers of Ludwig Edelstein* (Baltimore: Johns Hopkins, 1967), 247–301, "The History of Anatomy in Antiquity."

[4]A full account of the resumption of dissection in the late Middle Ages has not yet been written, but by 1316 Mundinus, professor of medicine at Bologna, was able to write a handbook for dissection of human corpses. It is perhaps fair to infer from this that the practice was regularly caried out by 1316. We can also perhaps push the certain date back to 1306 when Henri de Mondeville wrote his *Cyrurgia*. His drawings, especially numbers 4, 5, 6, 7, 10, and 12, which show human figures with the skin peeled back to reveal inner organs, suggest that Henri practiced dissection, even though he was not always terribly accurate at recording his observations. The drawings are in Paris, Bibliothèque Nationale, MS fr. 2030, four of them reproduced in Marie-Joséà Imbault-Huart and Lise Dubief, *La médecine au moyen âge . . . travers les manuscrits de la Bibliothèque Nationale* (Paris: Porte Verte, 1983), p. 99. There are also places in William of Saliceto's *Cyrurgia*, book 4 (anatomy), where dissection of a cadaver seems the only possible interpretation. For example, in

suggest that Benvenutus did in fact dissect an eye, or perhaps more than one eye.[5]

This evidence, inferred from a late recension of the treatise, is, if correct, the strongest piece of evidence we have that he lived in the thirteenth century. It is also worth noting that no physicians of the thirteenth century cite, quote, or mention Benvenutus, not even the Salernitans with whom he claims some affinity. He is wholly absent from the pages of Roger of Salerno, Guido d'Arezzo, Magister Gervasio, Francesco di Piedimonte, and many others.[6] His name and medicinal methods are first mentioned by Jean de Yperman in a treatise dated 1328.[7] If we assume that a person's theories and reputation need time to spread, especially in an era where every written document had to be copied by hand, then perhaps it is not stretching credulity too far to put him quite late in the thirteenth century.

These two pieces of evidence, the word *anatomy* and the possiblity of dissection, are not terribly strong, but they are the strongest available. And on their basis Benvenutus is usually placed in the thirteenth century, rather on the declining side of Salerno's great medical traditions.

Benvenutus is sometimes known as Benvenutus of Jerusalem, and one of the medicines in the translation is called "Jerusalem pills." In the

---

introducing anatomy to his students, he says: "et que cum sit possible anathomia seu ultimam membrorum diuisionem et eorum numerum ponere in scriptis, expositione tali tamen tedium perueniret quod anima de eius uirtute aut non aut aliquid aut modicum non utile comprehenderet. Ergo propter melius et utilius uidetur mihi ut procedam in anothomia ut promisi, uidelicet in communi, scilicet ponendo numerum et formam uel locationem membrorum que possunt esse sensibus manifestam — ut in eis cum incisionibus et cauterijs et operationibus manualibus absque errore procedere possis" (Oxford, Bodleian Library, MS e Mus. 19, f. 56vb, punctuation added). William died in 1276, and what he says here seems to indicate his usual practice rather than an experiment.

[5]See my "The Textual Tradition of Benventus Grassus' *De arte probatissima oculorum*," *Studi medievali*, 3rd series, 34 (1993), 95–138.

[6]Scalinci, "Questioni biografiche . . .," 201.

[7]Ch. Laborde, *Un oculiste du xiie siecle: Bienvenu de J,rusalem et son oeuvre: le manuscrit de la Bibliothèque de Metz*, MD thesis, Montpellier (Montpellier, 1901), 8, was the first to observe this.

Latin other medicines are also styled "of Jerusalem." For a time it was thought that such a name suggested his origins and that he must have been a Jew converted to Christianity.[8] Scalinci argues that he may have been a member of the Latin church of Jerusalem, but I think he comes closer to probability when he notes that the adjective *jerosolimitanus* carries a sort of magical property with it, like some of his other names for medicines: *gloriosissima, benedictus, beatissima, sanctissima.*[9] The fact that Jesus healed a number of blind people in Jerusalem (Matth. 9: 27–31; Mark 10: 46–52; Luke 18: 35–43) is perhaps enough to give the place and its name a special cachet for an ophthalmologist.

Scalinci supposes that the tone of Benvenutus's treatise is a teaching tone and that he must have taught at Montpellier.[10] There is no corroborating evidence that he taught anywhere, the references to Montpellier in two manuscripts being too late and too tangential to be used as evidence.[11] The usual sign that a manuscript has served as a teacher's lecture text is that the margins are heavily annotated, but none of the manuscripts, Latin or vernacular, is annotated in this fashion. Probably the only reasonably sound biographical inferences we can draw are first that Benvenutus was Italian and traveled, second that his travels indicate a peripatetic specialist in ophthalmology, and third that he probably lived in the thirteenth century, perhaps toward the end of the period. Other speculations, it seems to me, rest on shaky evidence and are not worth much. On the whole Benvenutus, like William Langland, remains another shadowy figure from the later Middle Ages.

---

[8]A summary of the arguments on Benvenutus's presumed origins in the Near East is in Scalinci, "Questioni biografiche . . .," 250.

[9]Scalinci, "Questioni biografiche . . .," 253.

[10]Scalinci, "Questioni biografiche . . .," 305–306.

[11]Munich, Bayerische Staatsbibliothek, MS CLM 331, a fifteenth-century manuscript, has a colophon that reads, "Iste liber constat in Monte Pessulano vi coronas." And Paris, Bibliothèque Nationale, MS fr. 1327, also a fifteenth-century manuscript, f. 37 (38), reads, "Cy apres sensuit le Compend qu'il ia esté ordonné par Bienvenu Raffe maistre et docteur en medicine qui a esté composé et compillé e ordonné a Montpellier."

The Nature of the Treatise

Where Galen deals with over a hundred illnesses that may affect the eye of a human,[12] Benvenutus simplifies: seven cataracts, seventeen diseases attributable to an imbalance of one or another of the four humours, two illnesses that may follow on from the last of the melancholy ailments, and finally a number of injuries affecting the eye. He ends with a brief collection of recipes for eye medicines and a diet recommended for those recovering from illness or injury to the eye. The work is organized, concise, and if not always wholly clear at least striving toward clarity. (All references in this introduction to the Middle English translation of Benvenutus's text are by line number.)

Although the treatise breaks no new ground and in fact rests firmly on standard medical assumptions about the nature of the human body and what may go wrong with it, no one has yet managed to find a source for all that Benvenutus has to say. Early on he quotes one authority, Johannitius, the name medieval Europeans assigned to the ninth-century Arabic physician, Hunain ibn Ishaaq. From Johannitius's *Isagoge* Benvenutus takes only the names of the seven tunics, the four colours, and the three humours within the eye. He agrees with Johannitius only on the names of the humours, and rejects the seven tunics in favour of two and the four colours in favour of no colour at all. And everything else in his treatise he seems to have set down according to his own learning, his own experience, his own sense of organization, and his own language.[13]

---

[12]Claudii Galeni, *Opera omnia*, ed. D. Carolus Gottlob Kühn, 20 vols. (Leipzig, 1821–1833), are not arranged so that all eye diseases occur in the same place. Vol. 20, however, the Index, contains listings under the headings "oculi" (and combinations with "oculi"), "oculorum" (and combinations), and "oculus" on pp. 434–439. The scattered nature of the entries may be evident in the entry "Oculi glaucosis," p. 438: "III. 786. XIV. 775. cura. XII. 802. ad oculos glaucos compositio. XII. 740. ad oculos glaucosos, quibus pupillae nigrae reddantur, compositiones. XII. 740."

[13]Scalinci, "Questioni biografiche . . .," 198–200 and 242–247, accepts Benvenutus's citations of Galen and Hippocrates as indicating a distant source, though Benvenutus does not quote either one and seems to cite their names merely as well-known authorities.

He is nonetheless medieval and traditional in accepting without question a system of physiology that rests on the four humours. A humour is basically a liquid, any liquid, and the four which govern the body's health are blood, phlegm, yellow bile, and black bile. Blood is associated with the sanguine humour, phlegm with the phlegmatic humour, yellow bile with the choleric humour, and black bile with the melancholic humour. It was assumed that everyone had within him a mixture of these four humours peculiar to himself alone, and this mixture produced what we would today call a person's health and temperament, what the Middle Ages called his complexion. Illness was caused by an imbalance in the humours, produced in a variety of ways, such that a person's complexion became altered with an overabundance of one of the humours. Medical treatment of all sorts, whether a herbal potion or phlebotomy or surgery or diet or whatever, sought to restore the balance among the humours, so that a person might resume his or her proper complexion and continue life in good health.[14]

Medieval methods of diagnosis included uroscopy or examination of the patient's urine; astrology, principally the alignment of the heavens at the patient's birth and at the moment of the onset of the illness; analysis of fevers and pulses; and observation of the patient's appearance and visible symptoms. Benvenutus restricts his diagnostic methods to the last of these, observation. The absence of both astrology and uroscopy gives

---

Benvenutus both cites and quotes Johannitius, but Scalinci passes over him in a sentence. Scalinci accepts the mention of a Magister Nicolaus as indicating a source, despite the fact that the name occurs only in the Ferrara incunable of 1474. That is, Scalinci seems quick to see a source, even where there is no verbal resemblance (e. g., see p. 246 on David Armenio's influence on Benvenutus), and equally quick to dismiss a genuine source like Johannitius if it does not serve his purposes.

[14]The ultimate source for the doctrine of the four humours is Hippocrates, whose theories are summarized by Galen in book 2 and in books 1–3 of his section on temperament (Kühn, ed. cit., 1: 492–694). Transmission of this doctrine to western Europe is largely the result of medical activities at Salerno, where Constantine's translation of Johannitius's *Ysagoge*, or commentary on Galen, was accepted as basic to further study. The doctrine is assumed, if not always explained, by just about every medical writer during the later Middle Ages.

the treatise a misleading appearance of modernity in comparison with other medical treatises of the same era, as if its author were sufficiently sophisticated to put aside such superstitious rot. But the temptation to see him as advanced beyond his time should be resisted: despite the inexplicable absence of some techniques, his methods, his assumptions, his treatments are thoroughly steeped in the traditions of the late Middle Ages.

In addition to the four humours Benvenutus also supposes that the brain has three ventricles, another assumption common in medieval physiology. The anterior ventricle receives all sensory impressions from the phenomenal world; the middle ventricle has a deliberative and reasoning function; and the posterior ventricle is for the memory. Some authors divided the anterior ventricle into two or even more parts, assigning to them not only the receipt of impressions gained by the senses but also a sort of memory of sensory experience and a common sense that filtered out physical matter from the impression before passing it on to the middle ventricle for consideration.[15] Benvenutus alludes to this cerebral anatomy only once at line 16, where he mentions the "fantastical celle." Fantastical celle translates an expression like "ventriculus phantasmatis," meaning the ventricle that receives and stores phantasms or images from the phenomenal world. We need not search out a specific source for this expression, since the scheme of the brain's physiology was widely accepted in the Middle Ages.

One other theory Benvenutus mentions has its origins apparently

---

[15]Galen proposes two ventricles to the brain, the cerebellum (the anterior ventricle) and the cerebrum (the posterior ventricle). The cerebellum absorbs impressions via the senses, and the cerebrum does everything else. See Kühn, ed. cit., 3: 663–670. Avicenna, *Liber canonum* (Venice, 1515), lib. III, fen. i, tract 1, cap. 2, discusses the three ventricles, their functions and interrelations. William of Saliceto even reports finding the ventricles: "Cerebrum namque molle est in sui substantia, causa < m > edullosum [ms nedullosum] habens figuram longam secundum longitudinem capitis, et diuiditur totaliter in tres partes: in anteriorem, mediam, et posteriorem, que partes uentriculii [sic] appellantur" (Oxford, Bodleian Library, MS e Mus. 19, f. 56vb). See also Walther Sudhoff, "Die Lehrer von Hirnventrikeln in texlicher und graphischen Tradition des Altertums und Mittelalters," *Sudhoffs Archiv* 7 (1913), 149–205.

with Galen and was current during the Middle Ages. This theory proposes that vision is the result of a combination of rays produced within
the brain, transmitted as visible spirit via the hollow optic nerve to the
eye, and projected outward onto the world of phenomena where they
encounter the natural light of the sun or moon or a lantern.[16] Benvenutus alludes frequently to this cooperative manner of vision. The first
mention is at lines 15–17, where he speaks of the visible spirit originat-
ing in the fantastical cell of the brain, coming down the optic nerve to the
eye, where it encounters the natural light outside the body. Elsewhere
when he mentions the blocking of the optic nerve, which he too takes to
be hollow, he has this theory in mind. Nothing in the theory seems to
intrude upon his ideas for the treatment of illnesses and injuries, but it
lurks behind his practice as yet another medieval assumption.

The treatise itself can be conveniently thought of as having three
parts: the prefatory material, consisting of a brief prologue and a short
discourse on the anatomy of the eye; second, the diseases of the eye,
divided into the cataracts and the diseases attributable to one of the four
humours; and third, the injuries and other miscellaneous matters. The
brief prologue (lines 1–8), made even briefer by the translator's tendency
to abridge the non-essential, is mostly an advertisement for the author,
claiming authority from both reading and wide practical experience, and
stating that he drew both together to produce this book.

What the prologue seems to indicate is a man who combines something of a university education[17] with something of the practical experi-

---

[16]Galen describes the hollow optic nerve in contrast to the body's other nerves in Kühn,
ed. cit., 4: 275–276. The theory is reported and elaborated by Johannitius to include the
projection of light from the eye; see Max Meyerhof, *The Book of the Ten Treatises on the Eye
Ascribed to Hunain Ibn Isha-aq (809–877 A. D.)* (Cairo: Government Press, 1928), 20–27.
The Latin translation of Johannitius says, "A cerebro autem procedunt septem paria
neruorum: quorum primum et secundum par ad oculos veniunt: vnus illorum est concauus per quem sensus visus fit et per eum animatus spiritus ad oculos tendit: unde fit
visus" (*Opera omnia ysaac* [sc. Hunain ibn Ishaaq] *in hoc volumine contenta: cum quibusdam alijs
opusculis* [Lyon, 1515], sig. yiiij-zij. The quotation is from cap. iij.).

[17]The Provençal translation calls him Benvengut de Salern, and many scholars agree. In
addition to Scalinci, "Questioni biografiche . . .," 196–200, the most recent scholar to place

ences of an itinerant specialist.[18] His university experience can be inferred from his having written his treatise originally in Latin, a language which by the thirteenth century normally indicated some sort of clerical education. He also refers often enough to Salerno, naming one of his medicines *diolibanum Salernitanum* (241–42) in its honour. Sometimes he uses a term current at Salerno, for example gutta serena for the first type of incurable cataract, where he seems pleased to be able to report the scholarly term: "The fyrst lechys of Salerne call guttam serenam" (282–89). At other times he prefers his own terminology, as he seems to do with the second sanguine illness, ophthalmia. He says, "Thys maner of infirmyte the grete lechys of Salerne clepyd obtalmyam, but I, quod Benuonucius, calle it torturam tenebrosam" (386–88). As a matter of fact elsewhere in the treatise he calls it *obtalmia*, but at least he indicates his preference once.

The combination of learned language and apparent Salerno affiliations with a specialty in ophthalmology suggests a man *sui generis*. His learning is apparent not only in his grasp of Latin but also in his pronounced ability to draw his experiences together and organize them coherently. It may well be that he witnessed or read about more diseases than he gives an account of or that there were times when he was baffled by a particular complaint, but he never lets on. He always gives the impression of knowing his art fully, competently, and coherently — and that his art is all there is to know about eyes.

---

him at Salerno is P. O. Kristeller, "The School of Salerno: Its Development and Contribution to the History of Learning," *Bulletin of the History of Medicine* 17 (1945), 138–194; updated, but with no change in Benvenutus's dates, in his *Studi sulla scuola medica salernitana*, Istituto Italiano per gli Studi Filosofici (Naples, 1986), 58. J. Hirschberg, *Geschichte der Augenheilkunde*, vols. 12–14 of Alfred K. Graeffe and Theodor Saemisch, *Handbuch der gesamten Augenheilkunde* (Leipzig, 1899–1911), book 2 (vol. 13), 248–255, rehearses earlier opinion that Benvenutus was a Salernitan but thinks the notion untenable (251).

[18]See Vern Bullough, "Training of the Non-University-Educated Medical Practioner in the Later Middle Ages, "*Journal of the History of Medicine* 14 (1959), 446–458; Nancy Siraisi, *Medieval and Early Renaissance Medicine: An Introduction to Knowledge and Practice* (Chicago and London: University of Chicago Press, 1990), 177.

This means that his treatise, for all its scholastic origins, does not savour of scholastic debate. He does not pose a *quaestio* (e.g., whether hairs on the insides of the eyelids are caused by an overabundance of phlegm), nor a *videtur quod sic* or a *videtur quod non* with other learned opinion cited. There is no *quod dicendum*, no refutations of the learned opinions of others.[19] There is simply a description of the ailment and a prescription for its treatment. Thus the extent to which Benvenutus shows evidence of his university education is limited, but at the same time the extent to which his experiences alone control the shape of his discourse is limited too. He shows a rare combination of the practical and the theoretical, the actual experience of dealing with patients whose eyes need treatment and the organizing intellect of a formally educated man.

But balance of this sort does not wholly characterize the treatise itself, for above all else Benvenutus is interested in the practical aspects of things. This interest is revealed early on when he discusses the anatomy of the eye (12–115) and reveals a limited understanding. Probably the fault lies as much with his source as with Benvenutus, though one does wonder how his sources could have been so limited if he was really at Salerno. His knowledge of Johannitius seems to have been derived exclusively from the *Ysagoge*, a brief commentary on Galen. Here Johannitius simply lists the tunics and humours of the eye, as does Benvenutus (30–37):

> Oculorum tunice sunt septem et humores tres. Prima tunica dicitur retina, secunda secundina, tertia scliros, quarta tela aranee, quinta vuea, sexta cornea, septimus coniunctiua. Humorum vero primus est vitreus, secundus cristallinus, et tertius albugineus qui est ante vueam tunicam.[20]

---

[19]See Brian Lawn, *The Rise and Decline of the Scholastic "Quaestio Disputata" with Special Emphasis on its Use in the Teaching of Medicine and Science* (Leiden, N.Y., Köln: Brill, 1993), esp. 66–84.

[20]Johannitius's *Ysagoge* is most conveniently found as part of the *Articella*, the medical textbook of the later Middle Ages, frequently reprinted. References here are to the edition of Jacob de Burgofranco (Pavia, 1506). This quotation is on sig. a3v.

11

There is just the slightest hint in locating the albugineous humour in front of the uvea tunic that the actual anatomy may be more complicated than a mere list of names shows. But where Johannitius explored this matter much further in his *Book of the Ten Treatises on the Eye*,[21] Benvenutus simply denies that there are seven tunics and claims there are only two. In fact in his *Ten Treatises* Johannitius had allowed for variations in the number of tunics—anywhere from two to seven, he said—but Benvenutus seemingly unaware of this nicety, relies on his own theory, though he does pay Johannitius the honour of adopting his names for the three humours.

In his *Book of the Ten Treatises on the Eye* Johannitius says nothing about eye colour, but in his *Ysagoge* he mentions the four colours repeated by Benvenutus: "Oculorum colores sunt quattuor, scilicet: niger, subalbidus, varius, et glaucus."[22] He also explains briefly how each colour may come about:

> Nigredo fit ex defectu visibilis spiritus, vel ex perturbatione ipsius; aut ex penuria cristallini humoris, vel quia plurimum recedit interius ipse cristallinus humor, aut ex humorum abundancia qui est similis albugini oui, aut ex perturbatione ipsius, aut ex abundantia qualitatis vuei humoris.[23]

And similar explanations are provided as well for the other three colours. Perhaps Benvenutus took his cue from Johannitius's fourth possibility, that a dark eye may be caused by the cristalline humour's lying deeper within the eye. His own explanation, at any rate, denies colour to the eye entirely and seeks to find the illusion of colour in the depth of the cristalline humour. He also tries to establish a correlation between eye colour, and hence depth of the cristalline humour, with acuity and duration of sight. This explanation seems more mysterious than useful to us today, but no doubt it reflects Benvenutus's conclusions from his experience. He is the only ophthalmologist of the period, as far as I know, to touch on this problem.

[21] Meyerhof's edition, cited in note 16.
[22] *Articella*, sig. a3v.
[23] *Articella*, sig. a3v.

The last bit of anatomy describes the three humours within the eye and distinguishes among them by touch (94–106): each feels slightly different from the others, the albugineus like egg white, the cristalline like fresh gum (that is, resin from a tree or shrub), and the vitreus like cooked lard. And he concludes with a description of the complexions of the humours and how they are nourished (107–115). Again modern readers may find these passages mysterious, but knowledge of the complexion of a given organ was important for prescribing the proper medicine. If the complexion of the albugineous humour is cold and moist, it will in some way be altered with illness — it may, for example, become cold and dry, and the change will be evident in a set of symptoms. Whatever remedy is applied to correct the condition should restore the lost moisture, and clearly the physician must know the complexion of both the organ to be treated and of the various treatments available to him.

The anatomy section of Benvenutus's treatise occupies 102 lines, about 7.5% of the total. His real interest lies in what follows, the illnesses and injuries and their treatments. He begins with seven types of cataract, four curable and three incurable (120–325). The definition of a cataract as a congealed water conceals its etymology. Galen calls a cataract 'υποχυμα,[24] literally "falling fluid," and the classical Latin *suffusio*, a pouring down, is a calque of the Greek. (Arabic *al ma' al-nazil*, falling water, is also calqued on the Greek.) Classical Latin *cataracta*, a rapid, a waterfall, was at some point in the medieval period substituted for *suffusio*, possibly by Constantinus Africanus in the late eleventh or early twelfth century. The condition was thought to be caused by a substance coming between the cristalline humour or lens and the external surface of the eye, thus inhibiting the passage of light from within outwards and from without inwards. The substance was thought to be a corrupt fluid, something that originated within the eye itself.

The four types of curable cataract are distinguished by colour and cause, and then the procedures for treatment, including the operation, are described. After the cataract has matured and the patient's brain has

---

[24]Kühn, ed. cit., 10: 119.

been purged in order to get rid of the excess humours in the head, then patient and physician sit facing each other on a bench. The patient is expected to cooperate to the extent of holding his good eye closed with one hand and keeping still — and this without any sort of anesthetic. Then the physician inserts a needle into the eye, catches the cataract with its point, and presses the cataract down into the eye's lower recesses. And he holds it there while he says four or five pater nosters, in the expectation that it will then remain where he has pushed it. The result should be that light will then pass through directly to the retina, without having to contend with an obstruction. It all sounds terribly painful, and no doubt it was, and primitive, but it is somewhat less primitive than it may appear. The technique of needling or couching a cataract was the only treatment available until well after World War II and the introduction of laser surgery and lens implantation. To be sure, the operation was refined and it was done under anesthesia from late in the nineteenth century, and bottle-bottom glasses were supplied to correct the distorted vision that resulted from having no lens.[25]

The three incurable cataracts are not, properly speaking, cataracts at all but rather blindness deriving from other causes. Gutta serena, the first of these, is now called amaurosis and is probably not the type of blindness from which Milton suffered (though his illness is also called "gutta serena") but rather a congenital problem. The second type of incurable cataract, with its greenish appearance, has been identified as glaucoma, though I do not know if modern ophthalmologists would agree.[26] The description of the third and last incurable cataract, the enlarged pupil, is too vague for us to be certain what its modern equivalent might be.

[25]For the early history of cataract treatment see Aryeh Feigenbaum, "Early History of Cataract and the Ancient Operation for Cataract," *American Journal of Ophthalmology*, 3rd ser., 49 (1960), 305–326. Contemporary treatment is described in Didier Fé lix, and Solange Leroux les Jardins, "L'évolution de la chirurgie de la cataracte," *Revue de l'infirmière* 40, no. 1 (Jan. 1990), 42–44.

[26]Hirshberg, op. cit., book 2 (13: 248–255), says that Ch. Daremberg, *Histoire des sciences médicales* (Paris, 1870), first recognized Benvenutus's second incurable cataract as glaucoma.

The illnesses Benvenutus attributes to an excess of the sanguine humour (331–569) are all probably varieties of infection of the conjunctiva, that is some sort of conjunctivitis. He describes six of these ailments, one without a name, ophthalmia, and four types of what he calls a pannicle. Classical Latin *pannus* means a piece of cloth, a rag, and in medieval medicine it came to mean a web, or growth of some sort over the surface of the eye. *Panniculus* is a diminutive of *pannus* and was adopted to describe a small growth on the conjunctiva, such as those Benvunutus mentions at lines 420–569. It is probably difficult for modern readers, whose symptoms usually receive fairly prompt and reasonably effective attention, to conceive of people who would neglect a furious itch in the eye until it had reached the various states Benvenutus describes. But in all probability the bulk of his patients had no regular physician, or no effective treatment from the one at hand, and had to wait for the itinerant specialist to arrive, an event that might not happen often in a lifetime.

After the pannicles Benvenutus describes four illnesses he attributes to an excess of phlegm (570–713). These are ingrowing eyelashes which penetrate the eyelid and scratch the eyeball, a poorly described growth of some sort that is covered with blood vessels and inhibits vision, a flesh-like growth upon the eye, and finally trachoma, an infection medieval doctors thought grew on the inside of the eyelid.[27] Ingrowing eyelashes and trachoma still occur today, and in third-world countries trachoma accounts for many instances of blindness. Benvenutus attributes two diseases to an excess of yellow bile (714–771), and both these choleric diseases are characterized by clouded vision. With the first the eyes appear normal but the patient sees what seems to be a shadow or a cloud between herself and the object she is looking at. The second seems to have not only the cloud but also some sort of growth upon the eyeball.

Black bile, the melancholy humour, produces five illnesses (772–913).

[27]For some early theories on trachoma, see Emilie Savage-Smith, "Ibn al-Nafis's *Perfected Book on Ophthalmology* and his Treatment of Trachoma and its Sequelae," *Journal for the History of Arabic Science* 4 (1980), 147–206.

The first of these is flying flies or spots and squiggles before the eyes. This condition is now thought to result from the residue of prenatal blood vessels in the albugineous humour of the eye, and most people have had the experience of seeing them at one time or another. The second melancholic illness is the sudden bulging of the eyes from their sockets. The third is an ungula or pterygium, a tumour-like growth that procedes across the eye from one corner. In Middle English it is called a nail (that is, a fingernail) or a web, and in modern English a pterygium, from the Greek πτερυγιον, meaning "wing," perhaps because it was thought to look like an insect's wing. The fourth illness is an itch accompanied by dryness of the eyeball, and the fifth is a sty.

One group of Latin manuscripts of the treatise ends at this point, but others add two problems connected with the melancholic humour. The first is an everted eyelid that may happen because of a badly medicated sty (920–50). Here Benvenutus imagines a sty on the lower eyelid which may leave enough scar tissue to cause the eyelid to droop, leaving the reddish underflesh exposed. The last melancholic infection, here called a muru or a wulgalpus, takes the form of a raw and rough patch between the nose and the eye (951–62).

The third part of the treatise is devoted primarily to injuries to the eye. The first of these is an account of how Benvenutus repaired the split eyeball of a boy from Messina and actually restored his sight (1011–18). This is followed by instructions for diagnosing and treating damage to the sight caused by blows to the forehead, temples, or cheekbones (1047–74). Then treatment is prescribed for a fistula, or boil-like infection, in the inner corner of the eye (1075–1142). Fistulas are again caused by a blow, either between the eyes or on the side of the nose. Since this type of infection produces pus, which may be taken for tears and treated wrongly, he follows up the account of the fistula with a description of real tears (1144–61). Next he tells how to remove foreign bodies from the eye, both fragments of metal or stone and the awn or beard from an ear of grain (1165–1212). Finally there is an account of treatment for a bite in the eye by a wasp or a spider (1213–35). The treatise concludes with several recipes for powders and collyriums and a very brief prescription for diet for those recovering from illness or injury to the eye (1242-1398).

Treatments

The treatments Benvenutus prescribes fall into four classes: cautery, phlebotomy, surgery, and pharmacology. Here and there in the treatise he refers to either a lecture or a treatise on cautery which he either has written or intends to write. This work has never been identified, but he does prescribe cautery for two different types of problem. The first can be seen in his treatment for the infection between the nose and the eye (951-62), where he prescribes first the excision of the infected tissue followed by a cautery in the wound. In this case the cautery may have had the effect of stopping a flow of blood, a technique recommended by several physicians.[28] He recommends the second type of cautery in the treatment for the second pannicle (474-505), where he prescribes cautery in the temples for an infection in the eye.[29] Here he assumes that the cautery will draw the infection to itself and then dissolve and heal it (489-91). As a method of healing the second type of cautery seems quite ineffective, but Benvenutus prescribes it fairly often.

Phlebotomy or blood letting was a standard medical procedure for reducing an overabundance of one or another humour and restoring the patient to the proper complexion. For example in the treatment for the

---

[28]See for example Guy de Chauliac, *Cyrurgia* (Venice, 1519), tractatus III, Doctrina 1 (f. 29rb-29va): "Quintus modus [sc. in curatione emorrosagie] qui fit per adustionem magis est conueniens venis apertis per corrosionem: et completur cum ferro calido." Guy cites Avicenna and Theodoricus as his authorities for this practice. Lanfranc of Milan, *Ars completa totius cyrurgie* (Venice, 1519), tractatus III, cap. xviij (ff. 202va-203vb) devotes an entire chapter to cautery. Among several objectives he notes the same two that Benvenutus espouses: "ad confortandum membrum cuius complexionem volumus rectificare . . . ad restringendum fluxum sanguinis." Bruno of Lombard, *Cyrurgia magna* (Venice, 1519), liber I, cap. xij (f. 87rb), also prescribes cautery to staunch blood from a wound: "locus cum ferro bene ignito et vehementer rubeo comburatur."

[29]Peter Murray Jones, *Medieval Medical Miniatures* (London: British Library, 1984), 98, reproduces from British Library MS Sloane 2839 a cautery man, i. e., a drawing of a man with points on his body marked for cautery.

17

first, and unnamed, sanguine illness, Benvenutus prescribes for a young patient blood-letting from the vein in the middle of the forehead (349–51), presumably to restore the patient's complexion by diminishing the overabundance of sanguine humour. And he recommends the same procedure for dry and itchy eyelids (865–66). Phlebotomy actually occupies a more prominent place in medieval medicine than Benvenutus's scant use of it makes evident. Veins that affected each part of the body were identified, and medical manuscripts often carry a drawing of the "vein man," a figure designed to show where the veins for bleeding lie and what part of the body they control.[30]

Surgery is perhaps the most accessible area of medieval medicine for the modern reader. Where cautery and phlebotomy appear to us designed to do things they simply will not do, surgery, for all its primitive nature, is at least directed toward an evident pragmatic end — and even in its crude state, it is recognizably the ancestor of modern sophisticated surgical techniques. Benvenutus is relatively sparing with his surgery, but where prescribed it does seem sensible, indeed perhaps the only thing possible. Surgical methods include the art of needling to cure a cataract and various excisions done with a razor, probably a smallish sort of razor with a pointed blade, designed for surgical use. He also uses two ordinary needles as a sort of slow-motion scalpel in the treatment for the first phlegmatic illness (587–94).[31] In all the surgical procedures recommended, Benvenutus carefully reminds his readers of the need for skill and circumspection in cutting: "so warly and so sotylly þat ȝe touche

---

[30]Jones, *Medieval Medical Miniatures* 120, reproduces a vein man from British Library MS Harley 3719. There are two vein men from Oxford, Bodleian Library, MS Ashmole 789 and from a manuscript owned by Irwin J. Pincus, M. D., in Linda E. Voigts and Michael McVaugh, *A Latin Technical Phlebotomy and its Middle English Translation*, Transactions of the American Philosophical Society 74, part 2 (Philadelphia, 1984), plates II and III (pp. 68–69).

[31]Jones, *Medieval Medical Miniatures* 109, reproduces a drawing of some medical instruments from British Library, MS Sloane 6. See also the many reproductions from manuscripts in Mario Tabanelli, *Tecniche e strumenti chirurgici del xiii e xiv secolo*, Biblioteca della Rivista di Storia Delle Scienze Mediche e Naturali 18 (Florence: Olschki, 1973). The difficulty with many of these manuscript illustrations is that there is little indication of scale.

not the tonycle" (629), "suttilly and discretely" (924), "so dyscretly that ȝe touch not the eyelede and the nose neþer the substance of the eye" (1113–15).

The most prominent weapon in Benvenutus's arsenal against disease is the medical compound, mostly herbal but some other substances as well. There are several varieties of these: pills and electuaries to be swallowed, powders and collyriums to be put into the open eye, and ointments and plasters for external use, usually over the closed eye. The pills are for the most part designed to purge either the head or the stomach, depending on where the illness was thought to originate. See for example the Jerusalem pills at lines 165–69, or Benvenutus's pills at lines 353–59, or pills of comfort at lines 813–19. The constant ingredient in the electuaries is something sweet, usually either honey or sugar, and no doubt they were pleasant enough to swallow. The diolibanum Salernitanum at lines 244–48 is an electuary, and there is a marvellous and precious lectuary at lines 690–702. The electuary mitygatif and aperitif is important enough that its recipe is given twice, at lines 730–40 and again at lines 789–96. But for all that most of the ingredients in the electuaries are spices to heighten flavour rather than drugs to lighten affliction.

The powders and collyriums to be put into the eye seem designed to produce two effects, either to wear away a film that has grown over the eye with some finely ground abrasive substance or to give ease to some other pathological condition. A powder like pulvis nabatis (515–23), made as it was chiefly of finely ground sugar, would indeed scrape away at the surface of the eye or at any pathological growth on it, and at the same time it would no doubt dissolve in tears and be washed harmlessly away at the end of the treatment. On the other hand, powders made of finely powdered beryl or jasper or pearl or crystal or sapphire (1242–59), while no doubt abrasive, could pose problems if they remained long in the eye. The collyriums (1338–79) also seem designed to scrape away at some growth on the surface of the eye, for they too contain sugar or a finely powdered stone as well as other ingredients.

Ointments and plasters see Benvenutus come into his own, for the most constant ingredient in all his ointments is egg white. No doubt egg white's appeal lies in its physical nature, for it resembles the albugineous humour. But the interesting coincidence for a modern reader is that egg white contains lysozyme, a natural enzyme found in tears, which has mild antibiotic properties. Benvenutus frequently recommends egg white on its own and in combination with other ingredients, and no doubt much of whatever success he had in healing injuries depended in large part on his frequent use of this substance.

And yet one must also admit that many of his remedies were either pointless or useless. The precious ointment of alabaster (445–56), to be rubbed on brows and temples to alleviate pain and to cure the first pannicle, would serve no purpose at all. The pills to purge the brain or the stomach do contain some substances with laxative properties, but in all probability such laxatives did little or nothing for the patient's specific complaint. The type of cautery designed to draw away infection and expell it was surely of minimum value therapeutically.

Nonetheless, the judicious restraint in surgery and the egg white dressing probably ensured a modicum of success. And two other circumstances also worked on his behalf. First an eye infection rarely spreads beyond the eyes, so the chances of complications setting in and killing his patients was probably limited. And second he was an itinerant specialist, that is one who treated patients in a given town and then moved on. Whatever failures there might have been he did not have to confront every day, and any public hostility or other difficulty over his treatments could always be met by getting out of town.

Manuscripts

There are four manuscripts of the Middle English translation of Benvenutus Grassus.

A Oxford, Bodleian Library MS Ashmole 1468

Pp. 378, consisting of three manuscripts: I, pp. 1–179; II, pp. 179*–298; III, pp. 307–378. Pp. 299–306 are binder's filler. Paper, some water staining on lower outer corners of manuscript I, some tears and cuts in manuscript III with amateur mending. Legible throughout. Watermarks in folio: Two unnumbered flyleaves at beginning show royal arms of England with motto: "Diev et mon droit," other half of bifolium: "DIVD" (neither in Briquet); pp. 7–174 a jug watermark, similar to Briquet 7826 and 7872, both from the first quarter of the fifteenth century; pp. 181–288 a hand with a wrist band initialed PB surmounted by a five-pointed star with a circle in the middle, similar to Briquet 10780, 10789 (lacking initials), and 10766 (lacking wristband and circle) all dating between 1524 and 1550; pp. 315–378 a mountain similar to Briquet 11662, 11663, 11664 (I was not able to see the cross on top, reported by Kane), perhaps a horn similar to Briquet 7666, other marks indistinguishable though present. MS I 295 x 215 mm., writing block 230 x 160 mm. with 42 to 45 lines in two columns; manuscript II 350 x 195 mm., writing block 240 x 155 mm. with 37 to 40 lines in one column; manuscript III 290 x 180 mm., writing block 202 x 123 mm. with 23–29 lines of alliterative verse in a single column. Binding seventeenth century, leather on boards, lacking Ashmole's arms, spine repaired 1959, modern gilt tooling on spine: ASH 1468.

Collation

Manuscript I: 1^{10} (wants 1–6, 10); 2–9^{10} catchwords, some signatures; 10^8 (wants 8). Manuscript II: 1^{12} (wants 1); 2–3^{12}; 4^{12} (wants 1–4); 5^{12}; 6^{12} (wants 6–12, 6–9 supplied by binder), no signatures; catchwords on every page except 191, 196, 238, 272. Manuscript III: 1^{12} (wants 1–4, 6, 7, 11, 12); 2^{12} signatures; 3^{12} (wants 1, 7); 4^{10}, signatures; cv is pasted in the wrong order, though its stub is in the correct order. Eight seventeenth-century flyleaves.

Contents

Manuscript I, pp. 1–6, Benvenutus Grassus, *De probatissima arte oculorum*, in English translation, acephalous, missing about the first four fifths of the treatise. Incipit: do we did nedill it after þe maner of agu-

21

lyng. Explicit: vouchesauf to ende youre cures amen explicit benevenu-
tus de jerusalitanensis.

Manuscript I, pp. 7–54, Guy de Chauliac, *Cyrurgia*, in English translation, acephalous, beginning in the middle of book I, chapter i, and
ending in the middle of book VII, chapter i. Incipit: be payntinges as þe
forsaid harry dyde. Explicit: þe whiche bene most communely leten
blode.

Manuscript I, pp. 55–171, a treatise on human anatomy in English
based on both Guy de Chauliac and Henri de Mondeville. Incipit: In þe
name of god amen here begynnethe a tretys of ypocras galyen lincon
henricus. Explicit: þat regnethe inne withouten ende amen.

Manuscript I, pp. 172–177, a collection of 31 medical recipes. Incipit: For to mak oyle of exciter tak calamynte herbe john. Explicit: and
gyfe hym tu drynke þis is prevede.

Manuscript I, pp. 178–179, a medical vocabulary, Latin and
English.

Manuscript II, pp. 183–247, a medical treatise in Latin, T and K
1204, unidentified, apparently a unique copy. Incipit: Qui bene ingerit
digerit egerit est bene sanus. Contains sections on measurements, sup-
positories, pessaries, clysters, syrups, ptissanes, powders, pills, electuaries, etc.

Manuscript II, pp. 251–297, Avicenna, *Canon*, book IV on fevers,
translated into Latin by Gerard of Cremona. Incipit: Febris enim est
calor extraneus siue preter naturam ascensus in corde.

Manuscript III, pp. 307–378, *Piers Plowman*, A text I 142 through XI
313.

Decoration

Red and blue ink alternate for large capitals and paragraphus in
manuscript I; some flourishing. Manuscript II no decoration. Manuscript III red and blue for beginnings of new passus; red for Latin
quotations, red highlights on initial letters of most lines.

Scribes

Manuscript I, one scribe throughout, a secretary hand, similar to plate 10 (i) in M. B. Parkes, *English Cursive Book Hands 1200–1500* (London: Scolar, 1979), first half of fifteenth century. Characteristic letter forms are the crossed and horned **g**, descenders on **f**, long-**s**, and long-**r** below the line, **e** usually has a horn, the body of **d** is pointed to the left and often horned, single compartment **a**. Manuscript II, one scribe throughout, a more cursive version of the secretary hand in Parkes, plate 20 (ii), having a larger, bolder appearance; probably sixteenth century. Manuscript III, one scribe throughout, an upright university sort of hand similar to Parkes, plate 17 (i), first half of the fifteenth century. Characteristic letters are the one compartment **a**, the short two-stroke **r**, ascenders and descenders do not extend much beyond the line, two compartment **g**, **n** and **u** not distinguished.

History and provenance

Kane supposes that the condition of manuscript III suggests that it lay unbound for many years. The loss of leaves from manuscript I suggests a similar fate. Probably first bound in the seventeenth century, though probably not at Ashmole's request, as his customary arms are not stamped on the binding, but probably aquired by him soon after binding. No other indication of ownership.

Printed notices

W. H. Black, *A . . . Catalogue of the Manuscripts Bequeathed unto the University of Oxford by Elias Ashmole* (Oxford, 1845), cols. 1275–77. W. W. Skeat, ed., *The Vision of William Concerning Piers the Plowman*, EETS 28 (1867), xxi–xxii. Thomas A. Knott, "An Essay Toward a Critical Text of the A-Version of 'Piers the Plowman,'" *Modern Philology* 12:7 (Jan. 1915), 130 (continuous pagination 390), describes contents only. Thomas A. Knott and David C. Fowler, eds., *Piers the Plowman: A Critical Edition of the A-Version* (Baltimore: Johns Hopkins, 1952), 24, describe briefly manuscript III. George Kane, ed., *Piers Plowman: The A Version* (London: Athlone, 1960), 1–2, describes manuscript III.

H1 Glasgow, University Library Manuscript Hunter V.8.6 (Young and Aitken 503)

Pp. 1–137, numeral 70 omitted from numbering series. Parchment, worn but well preserved, legible throughout. 178 x 136 mm. Writing block 108 x 86 mm. containing 15–16 lines in a single column. Seventeenth- or eighteenth-century binding, leather over boards, gilt tooled lines on covers, paneled spine, gilt title on spine: Graphei| de usu| oculorum| M.S.

Collation

Four paper flyleaves (i^4), i, 1 and 2 attached to boards. Two parchment flyleaves (ii^2). 1–8^8 catchwords and signatures (gathering 3 lacks signatures) a through h, c not used; 9^8 (wants 5–8) signatures ji-iiij.

Contents

1. Benvenutus Grassus (Grapheus), *De arte probatissima oculorum*, in English translation. On flyleaf ii, 2r in a later hand (18th cen.?): Graphei oculorum deus mss; and a second hand on the same page: Deus oculorum or of humane eyes by Benuonaus Grapheus. The base manuscript for the text here edited.

Decoration

Elaborate gilt and blue floreated initials with pink highlights, occupying the left margin and either the top or bottom margin or both, on the following pages: 1, 9, 30, 40, 50, 66, 72, 93, 102, 112, 130, 135. Paragraphus marks in alternating gilt and blue. Proper names, Latin phrases, technical terms in red.

Scribe

A single hand throughout, perhaps best described as a bastard Anglicana with a good deal of breaking in the formation of letters, giving the whole a formal appearance. Similar to Parkes, plate 8 (ii), last quarter of the fifteenth century. There is an occasional horn on **g** and **a** and final **s**, double compartment **a**, the descenders on **f** and long-**s** do not descend below the line, **g** is two-stroke with horn added, occasional hooked ascender on **h**, **l**, **f**, and long-**s**, as in an Anglicana formata; but the single stroke ascender on **d**, the three-stroke **e**, the final short **s** are more like a secretary hand. No distinction between **y** and thorn. Margins and writing lines are pricked and ruled in ink. Decoration and hand suggest a presentation copy.

History and provenance

On flyleaf (i, 3r) in the upper right corner is the price - 15 -. Same page in another hand: 9162. No other evidence of ownership or history.

Printed notices

Described in John Young and P. H. Aitken, *A Catalogue of the Manuscripts in the Library of the Hunterian Museum in the University of Glasgow* (Glasgow, 1908), 411.

H2 Glasgow, University Library MS Hunter V.8.16 (Young and Aitken 513)

Ff. 108 (originally) unfoliated and unpaginated. Parchment of second quality, defective in places, but legible throughout. 167 x 143 mm., writing block varies 127 x 105 mm., 114 x 102 mm., 123 x 114 mm., containing 23 to 25 lines in a single column. Original fifteenth-century binding, leather over boards, blind-tooled lines and stamped panels on cover, modern repair on spine now deteriorating, holes for clasps (now lacking) in front and back boards.

Collation

Two original parchment flyleaves, i^2; 1^8 (wants 8), catchwords. $2-6^8$ catchwords, signatures in 3 (bj-iiij), 4 (cj-iiij), 6 (bj-iiij). 7^{10} catchwords, signatures (cj-iiij). 8^8 (wants 5), catchwords, signatures (dj-iiij). 9^8 catchwords, signatures (ej-iiij). $10-11^{10}$ catchwords, signatures (fj-iiij, gj-iiij). 12^{14} signatures (hj-iij and d[?]j-iiij). Eight parchment flyleaves ii^8 (wants 2 and 3). i^1 and ii^8 originally pasted to the boards.

Contents

1. Benvenutus Grassus, *De probatissima arte oculorum* in English translation. Rubric: Of tonicle of the ey3en and the humours and cataractus. Incipit: Oculus anglice an ey3e is hard holowe rounde. Explicit: he wolde vouchesauf to ende your cures amen. Gathering 1, leaf 1 recto to gathering 5, leaf 5 recto, line 26 (= ff. 1–36). In citing and quoting from this manuscripts I have supplied folio numbers in preference to citing by gathering and leaf number.

2. Unknown author, *An antidotarie*. Rubric: Here begynneth þe book of þe antidotarie. Incipit: In the name of god amen ther shall be vij chapiter in þis booke the firste is of repercussive medicines (and after the summary of chapters) ther be twoo maner of repercussive medecines of the which some . . . Explicit: he regnith withouten ende amen, followed by a recipe for aurum potabile appended to fill the leaf. Gathering 5, leaf 5 verso to gathering 12, leaf 5, line 10 (= ff. 36v-96v). Another single recipe for aqua mirabile on gathering 12, leaf 6 recto-verso (= f. 97–97v).

3. Pseudo-Hippocrates, *The Book of Ypocras*. Incipit: This is the boke of ypocras in this boke he techith for to knowe by planette sykenesse lyfe and deth. Explicit: here endith þe boke of ypocras of deth and lyfe translate of astrolamyors þe best þat euer were founde. Gathering 12, leaf 5 recto to gathering 12, leaf 11 recto, line 23 (= ff. 98–104). The writing takes up only half of each page, one page to a zodiac sign. Recipes in a later (17th cen.?) hand on ff. 103v and 104v. For other

copies of the text see Laurel Means, *Medieval Lunar Astrology: A Collection of Representative Middle English Texts* (Lewiston, N.Y.; Queenston, Ontario; Lampeter, Wales: Edwin Mellen, 1993), 245.

4. Pseudo-Hippocrates, "Signa mortis secundum ypocras." Incipit: Here begynnethe þe tokenys þat ypocras þe leche wrote to knowe the seke yf he myghte be hole thorughe medycyne/ ypocras the goode leche sayde . . . . Explicit: he schall die of þe selfe euyll explicit signa mortis secundum ypocras. Gathering 12, leaf 12 recto to gathering 12 leaf 14 verso (= ff. 105–107v). Followed by a recipe in the same hand.

Decoration

Red and blue ink are used sparsim for rubrics and capital letters. No illustrations or flourishings.

Scribes

There are three principal hands, the first writing items 1 and 2, the second item 3, and the third item 4. Two later hands add recipes, marginal notes. Hand 1 is a secretary hand of the mid-fifteenth century, showing characteristics similar to plates 12 (ii), 13 (i), and 17 (ii) in M.B. Parkes, *English Cursive Book Hands 1250–1500* (London: Scolar, 1979). For example, the single compartment **a**, the heavily clubbed descenders on **f** and long-**s**, the single stroke **e**, the crossed **g**, the single stroke ascender on the **d**, the heavy ascender on the **v**, the ascender loops on **h** and **b** lean to the right, the whole having the appearance of having been squashed from above. Hand 2 is also a secretary hand with some Anglicana influence, about contemporary with hand 1, perhaps having a broader point on the pen. The general appearance is somewhat more squashed from above than hand 1, with thicker minims, ascenders, and descenders. Similar to Parkes, plate 12 (i), for example: two-compartment **a**, a looped ascender on the **d**, both Anglicana features; right leaning loop on the **b** and **h**, heavily clubbed descenders on the **f** and long-**s**, **v** has a hook to the left but lacks the heavy ascender of hand

1, **g** is a two-stroke letter without the cross of hand 1. Hand 3 is a somewhat looser, more current university hand, with some traces of Anglicana (e.g., the two-compartment **a**, the long descender on some medial **r**'s, figure 2 **r** also used medially), similar to Parkes, plate 17 (ii), mid-fifteenth century. The loop on **b** and **h** leans to the right, the **g** is crossed, the descenders on **f** and long-**s** less clubbed, more tapered than in hands 1 and 2, heavy ascender on **v**, the ascender on **d** is looped and the body occasionally pointed to the left, **e** is a simplified one-stroke letter. The whole has a squashed appearance, though there is more space between the lines than in plate 17 (ii).

History and provenance

No coats of arms. The flyleaf (i, 1–2) has a fragment of an earlier hand with a passage from 2 Chron. 27. Flyleaf (i, 2) has signature: George Blagrave his booke. Flyleaf (i, 2v) under a recipe (18th cen.?) is a table of contents in William Hunter's hand. Gathering 4, leaf 1 recto: signature Francis Sleigh (18th cen.?). Gathering 5, leaf 5 verso, partly trimmed away: Thom Garnett is my name; possibly Thomas Garnett (1575–1608), the exiled Jesuit (DNB). Gathering 12, leaf 5 verso, red crayon (18th cen.?): Charles Chancy; possibly Dr. Charles Chauncy (1706–1777), physician and collector (DNB). Last flyleaf (ii, 6 recto): Pedyr of holtworth estrologia. There are also astrological tables and formulae (16th cen.?) on flyleaves (ii, 1v-3r) and medical recipes (16th cen.?) on flyleaves (ii, 4v-5v).

Printed notices:

John Young and P. Henderson Aitken, *A Catalogue of the Manuscripts in the Library of the Hunterian Museum in the University of Glasgow* (Glasgow, 1908), 421–22, who mistakenly assign the manuscript to the fourteenth century. Laurel Means, ed., *Medieval Lunar Astrology: A Collection of Representative Middle English Texts* (Lewiston, N.Y., Queenston, Ontario, and Lampeter, Wales: Mellen, 1993), 17.

S London, British Library, MS Sloane 661 (olim 709)

Ff. 60; older foliation ff. 1–16 paginated 1–31; ff. 1–60 foliated 27–87; ff. 32–46v paginated 1–30; ff. 1, 30, 47 headed MS 709. Paper, restored on some corners, some staining, legible throughout, ff. 31–46 with printed margins. Watermarks: ff. 1, 2, 8, 10, 12, 14, 22 grapes, similar to Briquet 13073 and 13074; ff. 4, 6 obscured; ff. 21, 24, 28, 29 ewer with ornamental cover surmounted by a cross, similar to Briquet 12803 and 12834 (lacking initials); ff. 31, 32, 35, 36, 39, 44, 46 a large eagle displayed on a floriated standard with initials SIN, where the I may be an inverted F, Briquet 189, 190 are smaller and lack the initials but are similar in outline; f. 47 a wreath (?); ff. 49, 51, 53, 55, 57, 59 ewer with ornamental cover surmounted by a crescent, similar to Briquet 12853. 295–310 x 187–194 mm. Frame 261–280 x 139 mm., with 49 to 56 lines to the page in a single column, except for ff. 32–46 where 35–37 lines. Ff. 49–60 written on recto side only. Binding nineteenth century, half leather, gilt title on spine, gilt coat of arms on front cover.

Collation

Obliterated by the rebinding process, which has mounted each manuscript leaf on a separate nineteenth-century stub. Some catchwords on ff. 32–46, no signatures.

Contents

f. 1. Title page: Curationes Empiricae an Rulandi Praxis Medica an Ejusdem. Liber Johannis Pratt Sanitae et individuae Trinitatis Collegij socii seniori medicinae Doctor et Senior Bursor Anno 1660; three medical notes in Latin. ff. 1v–16. A physician's notebook, organized by part of body (head to foot), wherein the physician has recorded patients by age, sex, station in life, and treatment (usually herbal). Sometimes a remedy is given with no record of a patient. ff. 17–29v. In the same hand various recipes for herbal compounds listed by disease (usually in Greek) with a variety of compounds given corresponding to stages of the disease, vacuantia, auertentia, mundificativa, corroborantia, sistentia.

29

f. 30. A second hand of about the same time, four medical aphorisms copied from various authors: Hieronymo Tirayo (?) de stirpium historia lib 1 cap 130; Pros. Alpinus in libro primo de medicina Aegyptiorum cap x; Arnaldus de Villanova fol. 1030; and Scaligerus lib 3 de re poetica cap 16 (this last being a definition of a physician).

f. 31. Title page in a third hand: An observation of all sutch straunge cuers as hath hapned to my Hand since the yeare of our Lorde 1590 / by me Joseph Fenton.

ff. 32–46. Benvenutus Grassus, *De arte probatissima oculorum*, English translation, in Fenton's hand. The text breaks off after the description of a muri or wulgalpus, omitting about the last fifth of the treatise, the account of injuries to the eye and their treatments.

ff. 47–60. A fourth hand, a commentary on Genesis which begins with a page of comments on various ancient people like Plato and Moses. Beginning on f. 48 follows a lemma in English with a commentary in Latin. Ends with Genesis 24.

No decorations.

Noted in the unpublished Sloane catalogue, *Catalogus librorum manuscriptorum Bibliothecae Sloanianae* (ca. 1837), 126.

These four manuscripts are of two independent translations of Benvenutus's treatise on diseases of the eye. A and H2 represent one version, H1 and S another. I propose to discuss first the relation between A and H2, then that between H1 and S, before going on to comment on the nature and quality of the translations from the Latin. Finally, I want to say something about the textual value of the two traditions in establishing the text of this edition.

A close comparison of H2 with the surviving portion of A suggests that A was probably the exemplar from which H2 (or at least ff. 28–37 of H2) was copied. The chief reason for asserting this is that the two manuscripts are almost identical, save that A contains many brief lemmata where a word is more accurately copied, or a word which is not in H2 is included and clarifies the sense, or a phrase omitted in H2 appears in A to the benefit of the sense. Here are some examples:

A	H2
doctrine of cataractes [p. 1a]	doctrine of cataract [f. 28]
worshiping be to god [p. 1a]	worshiping be god [f. 28]
wex þat is attractyf [p. 1a]	wexe that is attractifi [f. 28v]
spirites and humours and woo and akþe [1a]	spiritus and and woo and akthe [f. 28v]
and so þey beten till the ey3e [p. 1a]	and the beten till the ey3e [f. 28v]
haue lost her ey3en [p. 1a]	haue lost he ey3en [f. 28v]
and þur3 þat many lesyn her si3t [p. 2a]	and though that lesyn her syght [f. 30]
But make a kerffe beside þe nose alonge in kuttyng þe hide onely and lete þat kuttyng be full litell [p. 2a]	But make a kerffe beside the nose a lete that kuttyng be full litell [f. 30v]
into þe ey3e and bynde it to with a lynnen clothe and and bynde it to another morwe [p. 2b]	into the ey3e and bynde it to another morwe [f. 30v]
as well of þe ouer lacrimal as of þe nedyr lacrimal and and þer ben two holes [p. 2b]	as well of the ouer lacrimal and ther ben to holes [f. 31v]
y-entred into þe si3t and ben fast and other hauyn ayenst sy3t and many atwene þe white and þe blaknes [p. 3a]	y-entred into the syght and many atwene the white and the blaknes [f. 32]
one handful and medle with hir halfendele þe white of an ey and medle in hem in þe maner of a plastre [p. 4a]	1 handful and medle in hem in the maner of a plaster [f. 33]
sarcocoll spykendard of each alike one scruple candi	sarcacolle spykenard one ounce of each rotis of

31

one ounce camphore mirre   fennel [f. 36v]
olibani masticia of each
alike a scruple and a half
rotes of fenell [p. 6a]

Apart from those places and half-a-dozen similar small variations, the two manuscripts do not differ from one another—even to the extent that where A makes awkward sense or little sense or nonsense, H2 dutifully follows:

> and yif suche be nouȝt [nought H2] ycured and ȝif [yif H2] þat [that H2] pece abide þere [there H2] any while on þat [that H2] tonicle of þe [the H2] eyȝe till þe [the H2] tonicle wexeþ white and lesith [lesithe H2] his liȝt [lyght H2] [A, p. 3a-b; H2, f. 32]

Minor orthographical distinctions apart, H2 is undeterred in reproducing a sentence with no principal clause. Both scribes also reproduce this phrase:

> Also þe [the H2] gumme doth [dothe H2] of soure plumme treis þe [the H2] whiche growen amonge vyne treis [A, p. 4b; H2, f. 34]

The verb needed to finish the auxiliary "doth" can be inferred from the context, but the point is that the ambiguity found in A is allowed to stand uncorrected. When an otherwise unknown substance called "anzoron" appears in A [p. 5a], the H2 scribe amends only to "anzor" [f. 34v]; and both repeat the same mysterious ingredient a few lines further on, this time giving "anzeron" [A, p. 5b] and "anzeroun" [H2, f. 35v]. It is of course possible that both A and H2 were independently copied from the same exemplar. But in most instances of this kind, each manuscript will exhibit a similar number of errors, and each will usually include bits omitted from the other. Here, however, the case is different: everything that is in ff. 28–37 of H2 is also in A, and A includes small bits omitted from H2. In such a case the probability is more strongly in favour of H2's having been copied from A.

Against this it may be urged that the dating of the manuscripts precludes such a relationship. But as I argue above, H2 has been misdated in the catalogue. Both manuscripts are written in secretary hands of about mid-fifteenth century, perhaps stretching into the third quarter of the century. In the letters **g**, **a**, **s**, **f**, and **w**, they both show resemblances to plates 454, 485, 565, 573, 595, 597, and 688 of A. G. Watson, *Catalogue of Dated and Datable Manuscripts c. 435–1600 in Oxford Libraries*, 2 vols. (Oxford: Clarendon, 1984).

Though too little of A remains to make an incontrovertible judgement, I would say that it is not the translator's autograph manuscript. No self-respecting translator would allow to stand uncorrected the careless syntax, omitted words, and the nonsense word "anzoron." It seems more consistent with the evidence to suppose that A is either a copy of the translator's autograph or a copy of a copy of it.

H1 and S, on the other hand, appear to derive independently from the same exemplar, which seems no longer to exist. Both scribes omit fairly large portions of the original, sometimes with a comment, sometimes without apparently noticing the omission. For example, in the section describing the eye diseases attributable to an abundance of the sanguine humour, there should be four types of pannicle described. Both H1 and S omit the last two pannicles, but only the S scribe seems to notice. He says, "Here my author left of to speake any further of the other two panicles. And beginneth to speake of the other infirmities caused of flegme" [f. 39v]. H1 simply goes on without comment to the diseases caused by phlegm. Another example, the H1 scribe points out a missing portion toward the end of the treatise, at a point after S has broken off: "But here it ys to be noted and vnderstonde that yn my Laten copy lacked an hoole chapytere, in which tretys of hurtys taken aboute the eyon, as by strokys of the forehede and the browys, the eylyddes, the boyth lacrymalles, the temples, and such oþer of their cures. And moreouere the nexte chapyter folowyng in the begynnyng lakked sumwhat, but not muche as I suppose, wher he tretyth of watry eyon and of teres, of corrupte humors lyke teres whych leches callen festeles" (1039–46). These omissions suggest that the exemplar used by both scribes was deficient in places, though the H1 scribe gives evidence of having once known a fuller version. None of the extant Latin manuscripts omits the parts omitted by both manuscripts, and we must conclude that the Latin copy from which the translator worked no longer survives.

Yet the similarity of wording in the two manuscripts leaves no doubt that both were copied from the same exemplar, perhaps the English translator's autograph. In the few places where the two manuscripts differ, the S scribe often makes better sense. Here are some examples:

H1	S
after oþer opynyon [p. 2]	after the opinion of the auntient phisitions [f. 32]
inocyon [p. 4]	incytion [f. 32v]
do hym sitte ouerthwarte rydyng wyse [p. 15]	do hym sitte ouerthwart a forme rydyng wyse [f. 34]
conseruyth [p. 48]	consumeth [f.39]
spere yn hys eye [p. 81]	close his eyes [f. 44v]

Yet for the most part the differences between the two are slight. S sometimes prefers a late sixteenth-century vocabulary (e. g., boulster or pledgett for H1's plaster, towe for H1's flaxen herdys). And sometimes H1 will include a phrase omitted from S, and sometimes vice versa. For example in relating eye colour to acuity and duration of vision, S notes "for those maner of eyes are oftener vexed with fluxes humors and teares" [f. 32v] where H1 alludes only to tears (74). Again in describing a fully mature cataract both H1 and S observe that the patient can see only light, either the sun by day or the moon or a lantern by night; S adds "a laterne with a candell light" [f. 33v]. And in describing the procedure for needling a cataract, H1 and S instruct the practitioner to lift the patient's eyelid with the left hand—and S adds "if yt be for his lefte eye" [f. 34]. On the other hand in dealing with the second type of pannicle H1 compares it to a freckle, "or lyk a frakyn" (434) where S does not. Again H1 gives the name of an ointment, "And thys oynement ys callyd preciosum vnguentum alabastri, the prescyous oynement of alabaster" (455–56), where S simply says, "and kepe yt to your use" [f. 38v]. H1 also includes a comment on where the second phlegmatic disease is prevalent: "And of thys sekenes we founde many mo pacyentes yn Tuscia and Marchia þen yn ony oþer contreys" (619–20), where S says nothing of the matter.

Differences of this sort suggest two conclusions. The first is that the scribe of S consciously updated the vocabulary of the treatise to reflect the usage of his own day. The second is that where each manuscript shows evidence of having been copied more carefully in different places, we must conclude that each derived independently from its exemplar. And since the two manuscripts are otherwise so close to each other in wording, we must conclude that they both derived from the same exemplar.

The scribe of S was moved to make his copy by what he perceived to be the plagiarism and numerous errors in Philip Barrough, *The Methode of Phisicke* (London, 1583, 1590, 1596, 1601, 1610, 1617, 1624, 1634, 1639, 1652), who incorporates into his treatise a text probably derived from the same exemplar as H1/S. In the right margin of f. 32 he comments: "This booke is moste of yt published by Barrow in his Method of Phisicke but he stealeth this, as he doth all the rest of his booke without acknowledging the authors and yet hath published yt verye faulse and left out mutch." Elsewhere as well he is severe with Barrough. At the description of the first phlegmatic disease, he comments in the margin: "Note here howe without sence Barrowe hath penned it in his booke willing to bind the needles at both þe endes, before you take vpp þe skynn" [f. 40]. Yet even though Barrough's text is faulty, we owe to him the impulse that produced this late manuscript of the translation.

Both versions—that in H2/A and that in H1/S—of Benvenutus's treatise were translated from the same tradition of Latin manuscripts, those containing the Standard Concluding Additions and the Standard Anatomy.[32] H2 eliminates the entire prologue, and H1/S abbreviate it severely. There is some evidence that the translator of H2 had limited access to a Latin manuscript with the Extended Anatomy, for he quotes

---

[32]See my "The Textual Tradition . . .," cited in note 5.

from it the explanation of the two tunics and the definition of the iris
(43–51). He also quotes from the Extended Anatomy a comparison of
the eye to a tongue, a comparison Benvenutus makes in order to prove
his contention that the eye has no proper colour of its own. The English
reads: "But for he hath none colour, therfor hit reseyueþ colour: as the
tonge lacketh sauour and it takethe therof sauour" [f. 2v]. This phrase is
not included in the text below because it leaves out too much of the sense
conveyed by the Latin, but nonetheless it does give evidence of some
textual contamination in the Latin manuscript or manuscripts used by
H2's translator.

There is no surviving Latin manuscript corresponding in every par-
ticular to either translation. The conspicuous gaps in H1/S, some of
which the translator seems aware of, suggest a mutilated copy, but no
Latin manuscript, not even those with a reasonably sure English provenance (BL MS Sloane 284 [olim Bernard 3650], Oxford Bodleian
Library MS Bodley 484, and Florence, Biblioteca Medicea Laurenziana
MS Ashburnham 225), reflects the necessary mutilations. Only four
Latin manuscripts combine the Standard Concluding Additions and the
Standard Anatomy: Erfurt, Wissenschaftliche Bibliothek, MS Amplio-
nianische Q. 193 (sigil Am); Forli, Biblioteca Comunale Aurelio Saffi,
collezioni Piancastelli, Sala O, MSS. 111/49 (sigil P); Vatican, Biblioteca Apostolica, MS Palat. Lat. 1254 (sigil VP1); and Vatican, Biblioteca Apostolica, MS Palat. Lat. 1320 (sigil VP3),[33] and since these
reflect the Latin version that is closest to the English, I have relied on
them to amplify or verify the translation where necessary. I also add here
a stemma of the Middle English manuscripts to make graphically clear
their relation to one another:

---

[33]All the Latin manuscripts are discussed in my article in *Studi medievali*. I have also
quoted from or referred to Naples, Biblioteca nazionale MS VIII.G.100 (sigil N); Vatican,
Biblioteca Apostolica MSS Palat. Lat. 1268 (sigil VP2); Regin. Lat. 373 (sigil VR); and
Vat. Lat. 5373 (sigil VV).

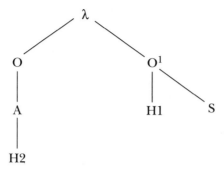

λ = a Latin manuscript of the tradition now represented by Am, P, VP1, and VP3.

O = translator's autograph

O^1 = other translator's autograph

Translation

The translations are generally good, in the B to B + range. H1/S are marked by two peculiarities. First they establish a distance between the translation and the Latin original, preferring the third person and producing what might be considered a report of the treatise marked by a good deal of indirect statement. And second quite apart from the conspicuous omissions, the translator prefers to abridge portions of the Latin rather than translate it. H2/A's problems can generally be reduced to a certain clumsiness in English, such that the sense is not always communicated. H1 begins by seeming to quote the author: ". . . yn the fyrst chapitre he declarith" (10), "Thus þan bryefly is shewid by this auctor" (24–25), "Consequently he shewyth" (26), "But Benuonucius varieth from hym" (38), "for as he seyth" (39), "as he hath proued" (39–40), "Now after he hath tauȝt" (116), "he consequently bygynneth to trete" (117–18), "He seyth that" (127). Sometimes when inadvertently in the first person, the translator will add "quod Beneuucius" (920) or "quod my autor" (963–64) or "quod he" (940). The effect of this is to suggest that there is not available to the translator a dependable set of conventions of translation. He conveys the sense that the first person singular and plural, as in the Latin, might imply that he was asserting something in his own right. Avoiding such assertion when he can seems to be a means of placing the authority for the statements with the original author, and of reminding the reader that he is doing so.

Although this distancing habit is frequent, often enough the translator simply puts the Latin directly into English, with instructions in the imperative and authority in the first person singular. This appears early in the treatise, in the section on eye colour and vision (54–92), and includes the phrase "as I sayd before" (86) without any attempt to explain that the "I" is Benvenutus and not the translator.

The account of the cataract illustrates nicely three phases of distancing. The translator begins this section furthest removed from Benvenutus: "And after hys doctrine . . ." (120), but two paragraphs on he is comfortable in the third person without reference to the author: "Thyes iiij spices ben curable, but neuer tyl þei ben grown . . . . And many lewde leches not knowing the causes . . ." (143–47). The instructions to the putative ophthalmologist begin in the third person because of an indefinite pronoun, "whoso," in the preceding paragraph: "Ffyrst he must porge his brayn . . ." and they continue, "And when he hath youen the pacyent . . ." (165–70). But they quickly shift into an imperative mode: "and sytte you also on the stoke . . . And with thy lyft hand lyft vp his oon eylyd . . ." (172–77). The instructions then continue straight through the operation and post-operative care, with the translator putting the Latin directly into English.

Once finished with these directions, however, the translator again becomes conscious of the need for distance between him and Benvenutus; he says, "Thys spyce of cateract is, as the aucter seyth,. . ." (225). This variation of distance characterizes the entire translation, as the translator puts himself in the author's place and says "I" and "my" without evident self-consciousness, and then from time to time re-establishes a space by stating "quod he" or "quod myn auctor."

When it comes to techniques for putting Latin into English, the H1/S translator avails himself freely of paraphrase and abridgement, reserving direct translation for places where the demands of medical practice make accuracy desirable. The prologue and anatomy section are abbreviated, but the section on cataract is translated with reasonable completeness, especially the part dealing with the operation itself. But once the translator is onto the incurable cataracts, the omissions begin.

For example at line 286, just after the word "spotte," the Latin reads: "et inter concauitatem oculorum apparet in colore serena" [VP1, f. 247v], a phrase of uncertain meaning but omitted entirely from the English. And in dealing with the cause of this type of cataract, "dicimus quod accidit eis in utero materno per aliqua corrupcione que dominatur ibi" [VP1, f. 247v], is not quite accurately rendered as "[it] ys causyd of a corrupcion of the moders wombe" (288). In describing the causes of the second type of incurable cataract the Latin reads, "ista egritudo accidit propter nimiam frigiditatem vel fragilitatem cerebri et planctum lacrimarum per nimiam angustiam et vigilias per magnum timoribus [sic] et uerberaciones capitis et per multa similia illis" [VP1, ff. 247v-248]. But H1/S reduce these causes to three, coldness of the brain, beating in the head, and fasting (318-19).

Elsewhere in discussing the treatment for the first disease caused by the choleric humour, a cloud or shadow before the eyes, the translator says simply to put no medicine in the eye but rather in the stomach (724-25). The Latin reads, "Ergo karissimi si oculi sunt clari intrinsecus, nullus puluis uel colerium valet talibus pacientibus istam infirmitatem quia si puluis esset corrosiuus coroderet totam tunicam et similiter si colerium esset violens excitaret reumam per totum cerebrum; vnde sic debet curar: primo purga stomachum et cerebrum de isto humore . . ." [VP1, f. 251]. Again in telling of the boy from Messina whose eyeball was split by a blow (1011-18), H1/S condense the account. The Latin provides more circumstantial detail: "Inter quos invenimus quendam puerum < in Messana > [VP3, f. 106v; omit VP1] qui habebat oculum incisum per medium et erat tunica saluatrix incisa, quam Johannicius vocat coniunctivam, et humor vitreus videbatur totus cum alijs humoribus oculorum. Et parentes sui adduxerunt ipsum ad me et nos curauimus ipsum sicud docuimus vos in presenti cura, quia intus oculo ponebamus de virtute a deo data et super oculum clausum ponebamus bombacem intinctum cum clara oui usque ad xv dies bis in die de virtute a deo data et ter in die super oculum de clara oui—et semel in nocte. Et puer recuperabat sanitatem sed tamen nichil videbat quia lux erat contracta [?] sicut habetis in tractatu cataractarum curabilium de primis paniculis qui accidunt ex vi percussionis" [VP1, f. 253v]. H1/S reduce all this to seven lines, omitting the repetition of details from the previous paragraph on how to use the medicine and tightening up the syntax on how the boy came to his attention. Nothing crucial to an ophthalmologist is omitted, and the account actually gains effectiveness from being more succinct.

Sometimes, however, H1/S add an explanatory phrase to gloss a technical term, and this technique can only have served to help a practitioner with his diagnosis and procedure. For example in dealing with an ocular tumour or pterygium, which the Latin calls an vngula, H1/S add useful glosses as the translation proceeds: "propter humores multos generantur vngule in oculo" [VP1, f. 252], and H1/S note: "a nayle, for it ys muche lyke a fyngernayle" (835–36), a phrase not found in the Latin. The description goes on: "et incipiunt crescere a parte lacrimali minoris" [VP1, f. 252], and the translator adds, "þat is to sey yn the corner of the eye to the ere-ward" (837–38). "Et cursus earum est semper versus pupillam" [VP1, f. 252] is glossed, "þat ys to sey to the syȝte" (839).

The H2/A translator's Latin is well grounded, but his English is often awkward and difficult to understand without recourse to the Latin. For example at line 97, the sentence beginning "Wherfore it is to vndyrstonde . . ." translates the following: "Est quedam concauitas in summitate nerui optici [blot] et concauitas illa est plena aqua <glaucosa> [VP1, f. 246; gummosa VP3] et diuersa est in tribus manieribus, scilicet in specie et in nomine et non in figura et in tactu. Vnde prima species est in tactu similis albugini oui, secunda est ut gumma recens, tertia uero habet tactum sicut lardum porci quando est coctum" [VP3, f. 97v]. The entire passage in both Latin and English tends toward obscurity, and it

40

requires some rereading of the text to determine that the *quedam con-cauitas*, "a maner holwenes," at the top of the optic nerve is actually the eye itself, filled as it is with its three humours. The English renders the sense of the Latin accurately enough, even "yellowish" as a translation of *glaucosa* is attested. (MLD s.v. glaucitas 2, p. 1081.) Perhaps the "Wher-fore it is to vndyrstonde" rests on shaky grounds, both of translation and of logic, and the doublet "in thre partis and in thre diuisions" for *in tribus manieribus* exemplifies one of the more irritating tics of fifteenth-century translating techniques. And in the last sentence of the same paragraph (105-6), the translator fails to translate the verb, *vocat* [VP1, f. 246]. Because of the awkwardness and the often ungainly English, H2 barely manages to render the sense of the Latin.

Similar awkward passages can be found elsewhere in H2. For example at line 152, the translator invents the word "accacioun." The phrase to be translated is *quia occasione predictorum accidencium* [VP1, f. 246v], "because on the occurrence of the aforesaid accidents," a phrase more or less clear in its context. The introduction of the nonce word "accacioun" may slow a reader's progress through the text, but the sense, such as it is, of the whole passage does manage to struggle through. Again at lines 223-24, in explaining why an iron or steel needle is unsatisfactory, H2 concludes that "gold most clarifiethe for his domi-nium for it is moste in his propriete." This is intended to translate *aurum magis clarificat propter dominium sui quia frigidum et humidum est in oculo suo* [VP3, f. 98v], a phrase mysterious to modern ears but intended to show the humoral sympathy between the substance of the eye and gold: gold clears the eye better because its lordship is cold and moist, as the eye is. H2 relies on the untranslated technical term *dominium*, which no doubt would have been understood, and the English technical term "propriete," which he seems to have misused (cp. OED s.v. propriety sense 1c).

In spite of these oddities in rendering the Latin, H2/A's larger prob-lem remains the awkwardness of his English, and that feature more than any other determined the choice of H1/S as the basis of the text that follows below. Just by way of example, note the etymology of "eye" attempted in H2 (punctuation added): "And the eyȝe is said of the senwe optico, that is said holowe; warefore, opticus is grewe and hit is said holowe in latyn" [f. 2]. The awkwardness can be explained: the translator is inconsistent in what he translates by way of etymology. He gives an etymology for the Latin *oculus* but explains it as the etymology of the English "ey3e." Moreover, he shortens the passage, leaving out bits that might make it clearer. H1/S simply omits the entire etymology.

Here is another passage, where the H2 translator describes the first kind of incurable cataract, the same text as that at lines 282–87 (punctuation added):

> Of the thre maner of kyndes that be incurable of cataractis, of the whiche maystirs of Saleren clepen guttum cerenam, anglice a shere goute. And these ben the signes of her knowyng: forwhy the ey3e appull ys blak and clere as though he had no spotte; bitwene the holwenesse of the ey3en appereþ in a shire sorowe, and the ey3en mouen alway with þe ei3eliddes as they were quakyng and as thei were full of quyksyluer.[f. 7]

This describes the condition, then called gutta serena, where the eye, though sightless, appears almost normal. Modern English prefers the term amaurosis for this illness, but H2's translation into "shere goute" ("shere" = shire, clear, shining; "goute," as in French *goutte*), though a recognisable attempt to find an English equivalent, does not make much sense. Also the clause "bitwene the holwenesse of the ey3en appereþ in a shire sorowe" seems to lack a subject and is otherwise difficult to understand.

Another example comes from the cure for the second type of pannicle as H2 attempts to explain the value of cautery:

> for fyre dissoluethe and drawethe and consumethe, and suffreth nought it to wexe croked on the tonicle; and that doth fire whiche drawyng to and dissoluyng and consumyng itte by cauterie; and that panicle shall be wasted; and claryfieth the ey3en withe medecyns i-added afterward wreten. [f. 12v]

The added punctuation probably does not make the passage any clearer, for the syntax is hopelessly muddled. Comparison with the text at lines

489–94 will reveal that the passage can be translated into some gram-
matical sense, even if the procedure recommended seems less than likely
to produce any beneficial result.

Here are some briefer examples of other awkwardnesses: "and that
with our cure, the whiche that folwithe, neuer after it worthe helpen ne
cured at the full, that they euer shall see wele after" [f. 12], where it is not
easy to see whether he means to praise or damn the medicine he is
prescribing. "Whan they ben feuerous and whan the feuer ys ycessed
than leuyth hym this vice of maladie, ffor they were nought well ycured
first at begynnyng neyther they were nought wele ykepte at begynnyng
from contrarious metis" [f. 19v-20], where the pronouns get a bit out of
hand. "Summe tyme for of ouer to moche habundaunce . . ." [f. 21],
where the conjunctions/adverbs are piled up to the blurring of clarity.
"For it comeþ withe moche sorowe and ache and with grete fernesse . . ."
[f. 24-24v], where "fernesse" may be a scribal errour for "sornesse" or
may be a word of the translator's own coinage.

As far as the quality of H1/S's translation is concerned (that is, how
accurately it renders the Latin), the most obvious thing to say is that
much is omitted. Most of the author's prologue and much of the anatomy section are omitted (I have filled the omitted portions of the anatomy section with selections from H2). Yet at the same time one must
admit that much has also been achieved. None of the descriptions of
symptoms has been distorted to such an extent that it is no longer
recognizable, and the recipes for herbal remedies by and large accurately reflect the Latin, given that the Latin recipes themselves show
some textual variation from manuscript to manuscript. On the whole a
physician of the fifteenth or sixteenth century could have done worse
than rely on this translation as a basis for treating his patients' eye
complaints.

All things considered, I have chosen H1 as the base text, with occasional readings from S, because H1 is the earlier manuscript and its
language more closely represents the daily usage of fifteenth-century
England. Where there are large omissions, I have borrowed from H2/A.

Dialect

The version represented by H1/S is clearly an example of a midland dialect, probably more east than west, perhaps even fairly close to London though lacking most features typical of Kent. In fact most features of the dialect of H1 can be found in the manuscripts analyzed in Angus McIntosh, M. L. Samuels, and Michael Benskin, *A Linguistic Atlas of Late Medieval English*, 4 vols. (Aberdeen, 1986), 3: 298–301. For example third person singular, present tense is invariably in *-eth*, *their* is usually some variant of *her*, third person plural pronoun is *they* or *þei*, *such* is preferred to *swich* or *swilk*, similarly *eche* or *ycche* is preferred to *ilk*, *many* rather than *mony*, *much* rather than *mich* or *mikel*, *be* or *ben* is found more frequently than *arn* for NE *are*, *shall* is preferred to *schall* or *sall*, present participle is in *-ing* or *-yng*, *sey* rather than *say*, *or* rather than *oþer*. The only unusual feature of the dialect is the plural of *ey*, invariably *eyon*, a form attested only in Worcestershire (McIntosh et al., 2: 262 and 265, maps 115 [2] and [5]).

H2/A is spelled somewhat differently but still seems to derive from an area near that of H1/S. Third person singular, present tense, is in *-eth* (or if after a vowel in *-ith*), present participle in *-yng*, third person plural object pronoun is *hem* rather than *þ/them*, present tense plural of verbs is usually in *-n*, the form *moche* is preferred to *much* or *miche*, *whan* rather than *when*, *ayen* is *again* and *ayenst* is *against*, the plural of *shall* is *shull(e)*, *yef* is *if*, adverbs end in *-lich(e)*, *yit* is *yet*, *ben* is *are*, *which* is preferred to *whilk* or *wheche*, *nought* is the usual form of *not*, the plural of *eye* is *eyȝen*. The preferred plural of *egg* is *eyren*, as in Caxton's well-known account, again suggesting a dialect area near London,[34] though the plural *hondys* rather than *handis* may come from further west.

---

[34]Caxton's story is in his "Preface" to *Eneydos*, in W. J. B. Crotch, ed., *The Prologues and Epilogues of William Caxton*, EETS OS 176 (1929), 108.

A Note on the Text

Abbreviations have been silently expanded, w' is expanded to *with* though the scribe prefers *wyth*; word division is modern; punctuation — including paragraphing — has been added. The H1 scribe often adds a macron over a letter and often finishes a word with a vertical flourish; in transcribing these marks have been ignored except in cases where the macron clearly supplies a missing *n* or *m* or *i* and the vertical stroke clearly means *-es*. Abbreviations normally expanded into Latin are here expanded into English, e.g., *li* is expanded to pound. Yogh has been retained except in those cases where it clearly carries the phonetic value of *z*, e.g., ȝucere, which has been transcribed *z*, zucere.

Otiose letters or words are enclosed in square brackets [ ] as are manuscript page numbers, and emendations are enclosed in pointed brackets < >. I have not hesitated to fill missing bits of H1 with passages from H2/A or, less often, from S; those from H2/A are printed in italics. Emendations (in the sense of changing a word or phrase for another) are kept to the minimum required by the sense. The textual notes give first the line number followed by a period; then the lemma from the printed text, omitting any pointed brackets, followed by a single square bracket, then the Manuscript reading from H1 (or H2/A as required). Where H2/A has supplied a portion missing from H1, comment is usually omitted from the textual notes.

Suggestions for Further Reading

There are two useful current bibliographies in the history of medicine: *Current Work in the History of Medicine* (London: Wellcome Institute for the History of Medicine, 1954-); and *Bibliography of the History of Medicine* (Bethesda, Maryland: U.S. Department of Health and Human Services, 1964-). Bibliography on specific ophthalmologists can be found in David C. Lindberg, *A Catalogue of Medieval and Renaissance Optical Manuscripts* (Toronto: Pontifical Institute of Medieval Studies, 1975). There are two general histories of ophthalmology, one on the science in general and the other specifically on the Arabic contribution: Julius Hirschberg, *Geschichte der Augenheilkunde*, vols. 12–14 of A. K. Graefe and Theodor Saemisch, *Handbuch der gesamten Augenheilkunde* (Leipzig, 1899–1911), which is still extremely useful despite its age; and Fuat Sezgin, ed., *Augenheilkunde im Islam: Texte, Studien und Übersetzungen*, Veröffentlichungen des Institutes für Geschichte der arabisch-islamischen Wissenschaften, Reihe B: Nachdrucke, Abteilung Medizin, Bd. 3, 4 vols. (Frankfurt: J. W. Goethe Universität, 1986), a collection of reprinted articles and books.

Other histories of ophthalmology tend to be either too concentrated on a single problem or relegated to a minor part of a more general history of medicine. I list the following in alphabetical order, but the amount of history each contains varies considerably:

G. E. Arrington, *History of Ophthalmology* (New York: M.D. Publications, 1959).

Juan Marube del Castillo, "A History of Dacryology," in Benjamin Milder and Bernardo A. Weil, *The Lacrimal System* (Norwalk, Connecticut: Appleton-Century-Crofts, 1983), 3–8.

Stewart Duke-Elder, *System of Ophthalmology*, 15 vols. (London: Kingston, 1958–1976), indices in vol. 15. Essentially a compendium of ophthalmological information, some chapters begin with a historical survey. E. g., 2: 3–72, on the history of the anatomy of the eye; 5: 3–23, on the history of ophthalmic optics; 5: 207–10, on the history of anomalies in the optic system; 5: 609–25, on the history of spectacles; 5: 713–16 on contact lenses; 5: 823, on the prescription of spectacles; 6: 3–5 on eye muscles; 6: 223–28, on anomalies of the ocular motility; 7: 462–79, on the history of ocular therapeutics; 9: 39–41, on inflammations of the uveal tract; 11: 63–67, on cataracts; 11: 380–88, on glaucoma, and 11: 505–6, on its treatment; 14 (part 1): 3–5, on injuries.

R. Rutson James, *Studies in the History of Ophthalmology in England Prior to the Year 1800* (Cambridge: Cambridge University Press for *The British Journal of Ophthalmology*, 1933). James's collected articles.

Renato G. Mazzolini, *The Iris in Eighteenth Century Physiology*, Berner

Beiträge zur Geschichte der Medizin und der Naturwissenschaften, n. F. 9 (Bern, Stuttgart, Vienna: Huber, 1980).

Stephen L. Polyak, *The Retina* (Chicago: University of Chicago Press, 1941).

Stephen L. Polyak, *The Vertebrate Visual System*, ed. Heinrich Klüver (Chicago: University of Chicago Press, 1957).

Thomas Hall Shastid, *An Outline of the History of Ophthalmology* (Southbridge, Mass.: American Optical Co., 1927).

There is a surprising number of Latin manuscripts of Benvenutus in print. Despite their relative inaccessibility, I list them here:

Giuseppe Albertotti, *Benvenuti Grassi doctoris celeberrimi ac expertissimi de oculis eorumque egritudinibus et curis: Incunabulo Ferrarese dell'anno MCCCCLX-XIIII* . . . (Pavia, 1897), extracted from the *Annali di oftalmologia* 26 (fasc. 1–2).

Giuseppe Albertotti, *I codici Riccardiano, Parigino, ed Ashburnhamiano dell'opera oftalmojatrica di Benvenuto* (Modena, 1897), extracted from the *Memorie della R. Accademia di Scienze, Lettere ed Arti di Modena*, ser. 3, vol. 1 (Sezione di lettere).

Giuseppe Albertotti, *I codici Napoletano, Vaticani e Boncompagni ora Albertotti dell'opera oftalmojatrica di Benvenuto* (Modena, 1901), extracted from the *Memorie della R. Accademia di Scienze, Lettere ed Arti di Modena*, ser. 3, vol. 4 (Sezione di lettere).

Giuseppe Albertotti, *Il libro delle affezioni oculari di Jacopo Palmerio da Cingoli ed altri scritti di oculistica tratti da un codice del secolo xv di Marco Sinzanogio da Sarnano* (Modena, 1904), extracted from the *Memorie della R. Accademia di Scienze, Lettere ed Arti di Modena*, ser. 3, vol. 6 (Sezione di lettere).

A. M. Berger and T. M. Auracher, *Des Benvenutus Grapheus "Practica oculorum,"* 2 vols. (Munich, 1884–1886).

Angelo Attilio Finzi, *Il codice amploniano dell'opera oftalmojatrica di Benvenuto* (Modena, 1899), extracted from the *Memorie della R. Accademia di Scienze, Lettere ed Arti in Modena*, ser. 3, vol. 2 (Sezione di lettere).

Ch. Laborde, *Un oculiste du xiie siècle, Bienvenu de Jérusalem et son oeuvre:*

le manuscrit de la Bibliothèque de Metz, MD thesis, Montpellier (Montpellier, 1901).

A. Laurans, *Bienvenu de Jérusalem, le manuscrit de Besançon*, MD thesis, Montpellier (Montpellier, 1903).

In addition to Albertotti's edition of the French version (above under Parigino), there is also an edition of the French and the Provençal: P. Pansier and Ch. Laborde, *Le compendil pour la douleur et maladie des yeulx qui a esté ordonné par Bienvenu Graffe . . . suivie de la version Provençale . . . editée par Henri Teulie* (Paris, 1901). There is said to be an edition by ? Masnow of the Provençal (Barcelona, 1967), but I have not seen a copy.

THE WONDERFUL ART OF THE EYE

1   [p. 1] A grete phylosopher and a profunde phycycyane clepid
Benuonucius Grapheus, after the sentence of þe [of] olde auc-
tors of phelozophie and of phisyk whiche he had radde, and
after hys propre experyence the wych he had by long conty-
5   nuance of his owne practik yn dyuerse parties of the world,
boyth yn hote regyons and colde, by influence and help of
goddys grace, compilyd and made a boke of the sekenes of eyon
and of her curys: and entitled thys boke and clepid it Deus
oculorum.
10   Of the which boke yn the fyrst chapitre he declarith what an
eye ys and the makyng þerof [p. 2] after < the opinion of the
auntient phisitions > and also after his own seying: a eye is a
rounde holow thyng, herde os the balle of the foote, [or as the
new scowrid basyn] ful of clere water, set in the well of the hede
15   to minystre lyght to the body by influence of the vysyble spyrit
sent from the fantastical celle by a synew clepid neruus obticus,
with the helpe of a gretter light mynystryde from withoute. And
conueniently ys the place where the eye is sett clepid the well of
the hed, for the habundance of watery humors and teris, the
20   whych often yssu [cum out] þer bycause sumtyme of sorow and
heuynes of herte, sumtyme of ioye and gladnes, and sumtyme
for habundance [p. 3] of superfluytees of humors causid of cold.
And forasmuche as euery naturall man hath such ij wellis,

11-12. the opinion . . . phisitions S] oþer opynyon H1
13-14. or as . . . basyn] not in any Latin MS

25 nature hath sett in euery hed ij eyon. Thus þan bryefly <is> shewid by this auctor what euery eye is.

Consequently he shewyth how an ey is made. Ffirst he rehersyth the opynyon of a gret leche clepid Johannicius and after he puttyth hys owne opinyon. Johannicius in his Ysagogys seyth that an ey hath vij tunycles, or vij cootis, iiij colors, and iij
30 humors. The first tunicle or cote ys clepid rectina, the secunde secundina, the thirde scliros, the iiijth aranea, the vth vuea, the vjth cornea, the [p. 4] vijth and the last coniunctiua. The first coler is niger, that is blak; the ijde is subalbidus, whytyshe; the iijde is varius, that is dyuerse in color; the iiijth is blancus,
35 yolow. The first humour is callid uitrius, glassy or like glas; th<e> ijde ys cristallinus, like cristal; the iijde is albigenius, like the white of an egge. Thus sayth Johannicius.

But Benuonucius varieth from hym in cotys and yn colours, ffor as he seyth an ey hath but ij tonycles or cotys, as he hath
40 proued by hys anothomie of eyon; þat ys to sey by <incytion> or kuttyng of a dede body. The fyrst cote he callyth "saluatricem," that is a sauyour, for it [p. 5] sauyth and kepyth the humors. <[f. 2] *Yif the first happeth to be broke or thorowe anythinge ys perforate, and for that hole may not holde the humors of the eyʒen,*
45 *warþorwe it seuwith that all the substaunce of the eyʒen is wasted and the eyʒe withe his humors ys consumed. The tonicle of the eiʒe ys that clere sercle the which to many it apperethe blak, to other appereth variaunce; and by the myddell of the eiʒe ther is an hole, the which hole is said "pupilla," anglice the "appell of the eyʒe," bi the whiche the visible spirite comyng*
50 *by þe holwe nerffe, hathe his outegoyng, and taketh lyght of a [f. 2v] grete clerte.* > The secunde tonycle or cote he callyth "discoloratam," þat ys discolurde or of no colour. Ffor as he sayth, in the ey of hymselfe ys propurly no colour, but dyuersytees of colurs þat

24. is S] omit H1
36. the] th H1
40. incytion S] inocyon H1

55 apperen yn the ey. For when the cristallyne humor ys nygh[t]
the tonycle of the ey, than the ey semyth of oon colour. And
whan yt ys in the myddys, þan it semyth of another colour. And
when yt ys depe wythyn, þan it semyth of the iijde colour.
Wherof he concludyth þat the ey of ytselfe ys discolurd and hath
no colurn propurly.

60 Tho men þat haue the humors lowe set and wythyn her eyon
semen blake and þei see best [p. 6] for a tyme, but when þei cum
abowt xxxti wynter or more þan here syght begynnyth to peyre.
Thei also þat haue the humers set aboute the middys of the
eyon, þei communly se wele yong and olde; and the colour of
65 the eyon ys meueable blak that we call grey. But often yt ys seyn
þat in þis maner of eyon obtalmie, þat is derknes of syʒt, and
panniclus, that is smale webbys, and oþer dyuerse dyseasis,
whych shal<l> be declaryd hereafter, thei grow rather þan yn
oþer maner of eyen colourid.

70 But þei þat haue humours situat or set nygh[t] besyde the
tonnycles haue eyen varied of diuers colours, and hangyn mych
yn whitnesse and [p. 7] hir syght is not right goode neþer yn
yowgth nor age. Ffor yn þo maner of eyon haue bendyng
humors of teris more þan yn oþer; ffor when the uisible spirite
75 descendyng down by the holow synews fynde aboute the tonycle
fresche habundance and plente of corupte humors, þei ben the
sunner disgregat and dyssolued from the humors. Also ys the
sight the feblere yn them þan yn þo that haue þer eyon meueab-
lye blake.

80 In tho propurly þat haue grey eyon the syʒt duryth better þen
yn other, ffor the cristallyne beyng resydent yn the middys
makyth the visual spiritys to [p. 8] abyde þere; wherby the
glassy humore and the tonycle of the ey ys kept yn, þat it may
not redely be disgregat and disparbolyd.

85 But yn þem that haue þer humurs depe downe, the whych

68. shall] shald H1

51

causyth the ey to seme blak, as I sayd before, better þan oþer
seyn for the depth of the cristallyne humor. Fro the spirite of
syȝt, commyng from the synew obtik, fyndyth the large space
and fulfillyth all the concauyte of holownesse of the ey ere yt
90 passe from the glassy humor and the tonycle. But os ys sayd it
dureth not in many to age, for comunly in thyes maner of eyen
ar oftener gen[p. 9]dred cateract and fumous syȝt than yn oþer.

And as for the humors thys auctor and <Johannicius>
accorde yn. <[f. 3v] *Ther ben thre humours of the whiche the first is*
95 *said albugineus for it is lyche the white of the naye of a henne. The secunde*
is cleped humour cristallyn for it is liche to the cristall. The thirde humour,
humour vitreus, humour glasy, for it is liche white glasse. Wherfore it is to
vndyrstonde that ther ys a maner holwenes in the ouer partie of optici
nerffe, and that holwenes is full of water yelwisshe and departed in thre
100 *partis and in thre diuisiouns: in kynde, in name, <not> in figure, and*
in felynge. Wherfor the first spice in kynde of felynge ys liche the white of
an aye. And the second as it were a fresshe gumme. The third hathe in
felynge as it were swynes larde whan it is soden. And alle ben in sub-
staunce and ben nought departed and ben in one figure, saue they haue a
105 *distinccion in the felyng and in name. Wherefor the first is that Johanni-*
cius albuginem, the secunde cristallyne, the third vitreus.

<*Of the complexions of humoures and of the sub[f. 4]staunce of whom*
they ben nourshed. Therfor y saye that the complexioun of the first albu-
ginosi humour is colde and moyste. The 2e forsothe is colde and drie, id est
110 *cristallyn. The thirde is colde and drie, that is vitreus. But netheles it*
hathe lesse of coldenes than of drinesse; for his coldenesse is temperate into
hete of blode, the whiche is in the eyȝeleddes, þe whiche is more nyȝ than
any othir humour. And sithen that humour vitreus and cristallynus ben
nourshed of the gummosite of the neruis, and the humour albugenosus is
115 *nourshed of the viscosite of the brayne.* >

Now after he hath tauȝt what an eye is and how it ys mayd

52

and of the colour and of the humors of eyon, he consequently
bygynneth to trete of the infirmytees of an ey and after of the
curys. And fyrst he begynnyth to trete of cateract.

120   And after hys [hys] doctrine a cateracte is nouȝt ellys but a
corupt water or a water congyeld lyke a crude, gendred of
humors of the ey, dystemperd betwyx the tonycle, and set
before the [p. 10] lyȝt of the eye and the crystallyne humor. And
of this maner of cateract þer be vij maner of dyuers spices,
125   wherof iiij be curable and iij uncurable. And fyrst he tretyth of
the iiij curable.

He seyth þat the fyrst of þe curable cateractys ys lyke ryght
briȝt whyte chalke or alabastre vele polyshyd and is causyd of a
stroke yn the ey wyth a styk or wyth a stone or any oþer out-
130   warde vyolence. The secunde cateractte curable ys sumwhat
white and lykenyd much to a celestyal color, and this procedyth
from the stomake and is comunly causyd of wykkyd [p. 11]
metis, wherof a groos fumosytee resoluyd ascendyth vp ynto the
brayn and from thens fallyth downe into the eyon. The thyrde
135   cateractte curable ys also whytyshe but it turnyth into the color
of ashes and is comunly gendrid of the payn of the hede, as the
mygrym and such other, and is causid of gret sorowe sumtyme
and of grete heuynes cawsyng grette wepyng, and sumtyme of
much colde and much watche and such oþer. And the iiijth spice
140   of cateracct curable ys of sytrynne color and it ys comunly
gendryd of exces meete and drynk yndegest, and also of gret
labour and sumtyme humurs [p. 14] malencoly.

Thyes iiij spices ben curable, but neuer tyl þei ben grown and
confermed with his signe; and the tokyn of hyr complexion or
145   confermyng is when the pacyent seyth ryȝth nowght but yf it be
bryȝtnes of the sunne by day or the mone by nyȝt or a lanterne.
And many lewde leches not knowyng the causes nor propertes

132-42. H1 p. 12 is blank; p. 13 repeats p. 11; a later hand (17th century?) in lower
margin of p. 11 remarks: "after this page yow follow to the 14. page"

of thyes maner of cateracties weyn to cure þem with purgacions, powders, and plastrys, but thei be disceyuyd. <[f. 5] *Forwhy* 150 *thoo cataractes ben vndyr the tonicles of the eyʒen and ben engendred of humours of the eyʒen, that is the humour albuginoys. Fforwhy thorugh accacioun of the forsaid causes, the humour albuginoys ys dissoluid in partye and hit rotith; and that roted is as it were water congelid and crudded. And it is putten afore the lyght and afore the eyʒe appill, bitwene* 155 *the tonicle and the cristallyne humour; the which the Sarazyns and the Arabies clepen hit "amesarca," that is in Latyn "aqua putrefacta," in Englisshe "water yroted" in the eyʒe. Of the whiche it sheweth openly that they mowen nought be holpon withe poudres neither with other medecyns yputte in the eyʒe, sithen the mater and all the humours of the eyʒen withyn* 160 *the tonicles ben conteyned.* > For thyes maner of diseasys may not be curid oonly by medycyns, neyther ynward or outwarde nor princypally, but by thys craft that ys callyd "ars acuaria," [p. 15] that ys to saye the craft of nedyl. In whych craft whoso wyll procede artyfycyally he must begyn thus:

165 Ffyrst he must porge his brayn with pelett callyd pillule Iherosolimitane, wherof thus is the makyng: Take turbite, aloes, epatica — of euerych an ownce; macys, quibybus, mastic, and dylle — of eche of þem a dram. And beete þem into pouder and confecte þem with the jows of rose, and make þerof pelatis.

170 And when he hath youen the pacyent purgacioun, on the day next foloyng abowt ix of the clok whyle he is fastyng do hym sitte ouerthwart <a forme>, rydyng-wyse; and sytte you also on the stoke yn lyk wyse face to face. And do the pacyent [p. 16] to holde the hole eye cloos with hys oon hande, and charge hym 175 that he syt stydfastly styl and styre not. And þen blysse the and begyn thy craft in the name of Ihesu Cryste.

And with thy lyft hand lyft vp hys oon eylyd, and with þin oþer hande put yn thy nedyl made þerfore on the forþer syde from the nose. And softly thyrl the tonycle saluatrice, and alwey

172. a forme S] omit H1

180   wryth thy fyngers too and fro tyll þou touche wyth the poynt the
corupte water, the whych ys the cateracte. And then begyn to
remeue downward from aboue wyth the poynte the sayd corrupte water fro beforne the syȝth, and dryue yt down beneth [p.
17] and þere kepe it styl with the poynt of the nedyl as long as
185   þou mayst say iij or iiij tymes "pater noster."

    Than remeue esely the nedyl therfro. And it hape to ryse vp
ayen, bryng it down ageyne to the corner of the ey to the ere-
warde. But here beware þat after tyme the nedyl hath towchyd
the cateract þou schalt no more wrythe thy fyngers to and fro tyl
190   þat it be set yn hys place as it ys seyd before. And þan softlye
drawe out thy nedyl as þou put it yn, alway thyrllyng thy
fingurs to and fro tyl yt be all owte.

    And anon make a plaster of coton or of flaxe herdis [p. 18]
with the whyte of an egg and ley it on the [the] sore eye. And do
195   hym lye down in hys bed wyde opon ix days. After charge hym
that he ster not hys eye all that tyme. And thryys yn the day and
tryys yn the nyght, remeue the playster. And he to [to] lye yn a
derke house. And for hys dyet the ix days, lete hym ete rere
eggis wyth breed. And yf he be yong and strong, lete hym
200   drynk water; and yf he be yn age, lete hym drynk wyne medlyd
water. Som byd hym ete fresch flesche and hennys, but we
forbedde yt, for þei be noryshyng of mych blode — ther myght
be gendryd yn the eyon that [p. 19] myȝte be contrary to oure
cure.
205   When the ix days ar past, make on the eye a tokyne of the
crosse and let hym ryse vp and wasche wele hys face and hys
eyon wyth fayr colde water. And after that doo hys occupacion
that he hath to doon. And in thys wyse be curyd all the caterac-
tis curable, and who that wyll cure hem oþerwyse shall dyseyue
210   þemselfe, ignorant of the true craft of curyng.

    And thys crafte aforesayde ys callyd the nedyll crafte, for it ys
excercysed and don with the nedyll. But alway beware that the
nedyll be of golde or of syluer or of clene [p. 20] Spanesh laten,

215

and yn no wyse of yren nor of stele. And þat ys for the hardnesse þat dyssoluyth suche as yt towchyth. Another cause ys for yf the cateract be harde yn drawyng down therof, the poynt myȝte lyȝtely breke, for yron and stele arne frayle and brytyll, and so the poynt abydyng yn the eye myȝte cause < a > consumpcion of the eye thorugth habundance of terys and gretnese of payne.

220

< [f. 6v] *The third forsoth the nedill of yren more greuethe and more weyȝth, and the pacient felithe his hardenes more than it were of siluer or of golde. But of siluer or of golde boþe ben full good for her clennes and her softenes, but golde moste clarifiethe for his dominium for it is moste in his propriete.* >

225

Thys spyce of cateract is, as the aucter seyth, easely and sone cured. But yit þei þat ben cured seen not ryght wele, forasmuch as the [p. 21] humor yn the eye ys yn party dysgregat and dyssoluyd by the stroke and be bruser therof, whych stroke was cause of the cateract.

230

The secunde spyce of cateract curable, yf it be welle cured with the nedyl as it is seyd before, the lyȝte turneth ayen to hys fyrst brygh < t > nes, for by purenes of the humurs whych be not dyssolued and also for habundance of the vysible spyrit yn the eye. And therfore tho þat be cured of thyes maner of cateract

235

[seen better þan oþer that be cured of this cataracte] see better after then those that be cured of the other cataracte caused of a strook or outward blowe.

The thyrde spyce of cateract curable after that yt ys cured with the nedyl and the syght recouered, yf it dure not long yn

240

[p. 22] that astate < then let > it be holpen with oþer medicynes, as with oure electuarie that we call diolibanum Salernitanum and wyth good dyet as yt schal be tolde after. The makyng of oure diolibanum ys thys:

218. a S] of H1
232. bryghtnes] bryghnes H1
240. then let S] lesse þan H1

Take olibanum ij vncys; clouys, notemygys, notys of Indie,
245   saferon, of eche lyke — that ys of ycche a dram and an halfe; of
good castor a dram. Bete all thyes to powder and sars þem and
confete hem togedder wyth claryfyed hony, and make electuarye. And of thys lete the pacyent resceyue yn the mornyng
fastyng the quantite of a good chasteyn or of a walnot, and [p.
250   23] at eue to bed-ward as much. And for hys dyet <let him>
vsyn dygestyble metys hote and moyst, whych engender good
blode. And let hym beware of contrarius metys, and for cowes
fleshe, ghetys fleshe, and eelys, and such oþer, and specyally of
rawe onyons, for they be specyally contrarius, as I have prouyd
255   be experyence. Ffor many haue come too me with cateractys
not fully confermede: I made hem, quod he, to ete rawe onyons
to conferme with the cateract, and they were sone spede. Wherfore, rawe onyons be noyows to the syȝte. And yn wynter lett
nat the pacyent drynk hoote wynes [p. 24] yn whych be put
260   sawge and rewe. And abstene he from commenyng of women,
nor let nat hym com in no bath nor stew. And yff he wyll
algattis bath hym, lete hym enter to a stewe or fat wyth the
water of the decoccion of camamyl or oþer swete smellyng
herbys, but lett hym kepe hys hede without the wessyl þat the
265   fume cum not ynto hys eyon, for þat were noyous. The forsayd
electuarye of diolibanum Salernitanum ys also good, as he
seyth, to avoyde terys and to dystroye þem. And so yt ys also for
al maner payne of the mygryme that ys caused of flume.

The iiijth spyce of [p. 25] cateract curable, þat ys of colour
270   cityrne, ys herder þan any of the oþer and also yt ys rownd.
Wherfore yt may not be leyd ryght downe yn the ey, for yt wyl
not abyde þere for the rowndnesse and hardnes þereof. And
þerefore yt must be leyd yn the corner of the ey to the ere-
warde, and þere be kepte with the nedyll a good whyle as yt ys
275   beforeseyd.

250. let him S] þat ye H1

But hyer fynyally I wyl ȝe knowe, ȝe þat wyll be practyfe yn
the acurye crafte, þat noon of þies iiij curable cateractes yt
nedyth to doon from clene metys abstynence, as I haue prouyd
by experyence, [p. 26] saue oonly yn the thyrde spyce, where
280   neuerthelesse yt behouyth alwey to haue confortatiuus and neutrytyuus of the vysible spiryt yn the eyon.

The iij cateractes vncurable be thyes: The fyrst lechys of
Salerne call guttam serenam, and thys ys the sygne of knowyng:
The pyupyl of the ey, þat ys place yn the myddys of the eye
285   where ys the resydence of the syȝte, ys blake and clere as towe yt
hade no spotte, and the ey ys meuyng alwey with the lyddys
tremelyng as tow þei were ful of quyksyluer. And thys cateract
[p. 27] ys causyd of a corrupcion of the moders wombe. And
þerfore tho comunly that haue thys cateracte byth blynde borne,
290   off whom, quod he, I haue assayd with dyuerse medycyns to
cure many, but yt wolde neuer be: I cowd neuer heer þat ony
such was cured. But nat forþan I perceuyd wele þat of thies
maner cateractys were dyuersytee, ffor sum of them myȝte see
the bryȝtnes of the son and went be the way wyth opon ey as
295   thow þei had perfyȝtly seyn. And sum myȝte see the stature of a
man and of a best or of another thyng and not els. And [p. 28]
sum had thys lytle parte of lyȝte to her lyues ende, and of sum yt
vanyshyd avaye and þei hade no more syȝte as towe þei neuer
had none. <[f. 7v] *Wherefore yif me yeue all the golde of the worlde*
300   *and all the leches thorugh trauailled ther, none of hem with no medecyn*
may helpe but oure lorde Jhesu Crist thorow his vertue.> Wherfor I
wyll that ye knowe all thyes maner of cateractes ben vncurable,
lesse þan God cure þem, ffor the neruys obtyk be so opylate,
that ys such maner of synewes ben so stoppyd and mortifyed,
305   þat no medycyn may helpe yt. And þerfor thyes cateractys we
clepyn guttam serenam, ffor yt ys gendyrde of a corrupcion
commyng downe from the brayn yn the maner of a drope of
water whych corruptyth and dyssol[p. 29]uyth all the humurs of
the ey; that fro thens foreward the concaue or the holow syn-

58

310 ewys be so stoppyd and ouerlayd that the vysyble spiryte may
no more passe down by them.

The secunde maner of cateractys vncurable ys the whych
apperyth withyn the ey of grene color, lyke water stondyng yn
watry placys not much meuyd nor renewed. <[f. 8] *Wherfor*
315 *kno<w> well that this maner of cataractes comethe into the eyȝen litell*
and lytell, but it comethe sodenly so fro that houre forward he seithe no
more. > And thys cateracte ys the worst of all oþer and ys gendred and causyde of ouermych coldnes of the brayn, of gret
betyng yn the hede, fer fastyng, and such other.
320 The thyrde vncurable cateracte ys when the pupil [p. 30] ys
dylated and sprede abroode so fer that no cerkyl may be seyn
withyn the tonycle. [any of thyes iij labourth yn veynne] <*But*
all the naterall lyght after that it is so spredde abrode that none helpe may
helpe hem that longethe to the medecyne. > <And whoso laboreth to
325 cuer any of these 3 cataractes doth losse his labor. >

Now after the doctryne and knowlege of cateractes and the
nombre of them, and whych be curable and whych nat, and the
cures of the curable and the knowlege of the causes of
vncurable — now I wyll, quod he, speke of oþer sekenes causyd
330 and occasyonyd of the iiij humors, as blode, flewme, color, and
malyncolye. But first of the sekenes causyd of blode, for often-
tymes [p. 31] for multitude of blode þer growyth a rednes yn the
ey with a grete brynnyng, and after yt tornyth into grete ycche.
And thys dysease makyth the here of the eylyddys to fall awey,
335 and of many yt semyth of non here. And yf thys sekenes be nat
curyd in a yere, yt wyll make the eyelyddys to turne vp and
make the pacyent bleryed. Wherfor ere yt cum to the poynt, yt
may be curyd, quod he, with my colery that ys clepyd colerium
Iherosolimitanum that ys mayd yn thyse wyse:
340 Take tutie of Alexandrye an vnce and beyt to smale powder,

315. know] knowell H2
324–25. And who so . . . labor S] omit H1

and temper yt with ij pounds [p. 32] of whyte wyne, þat ys a
quarte. And put yt yn a new erthyn pote, and put þerto an vnce
of dry roses and boyl yt wyth a sokyng fyre tyl the wyne be half
wasted. Then clense yt through[t] a lynnyn cloyth and kepe yt
345   yn a vyall of glas. And morn and yeuen put yt ynto hys eyon.
And yf yt be takyn betymes, the pacyent schal be curyd withyn
a weke or ij at moost. And wyth thys, quod he, I haue holpyn
manny.

Neuerthelesse, or the practyser begyn, lete hym make the
350   pacyent, yf he be yong, to blede on the veyne yn the myddys of
the [p. 33] hede. Yf he be agyd, purge hys brayne wyth pullyalys or pelatys made ayen ycche, thus made:

Take aloes, epatyk, sandalys rubeus, esule, rubarbe ana half
an vnce; turbit, catapucie minoris, and agaryk ana a quarteron
355   of an vnce; and confect hem with the jus of mugworte. And lete
the pacyent resceyue therof after þeir strength. And truly þies
peletys ar not good only for ycche of eyon, but also for all maner
ycche and skabe of what humor þat euer yt be causyd. And thies
arn clepyd pillule Benuenuci.

360   Also ther ben other sekenes of eyon causyd and engendrede
[p. 34] of blode, as obtalmies and panniculus. And thyes happyn to be engendred more abowte the ende of August and so
forth to the ende of Septembre more thanne oþer tymes of the
yere, for bycause of chaungyng of the eyre. Obtalmies comunly
365   haue þer domyne or power þat tyme for bycause of dyuersytees
of frutees þat be eten at that tyme, and by occasyon of obtalmyes be founde yn the eye pannycles.

Than yt ys conuenyent to tell what ys obtalmye and what ys a
pannycle. Obtalmye ys a corrupte blode gendryd of hote
370   humurs, and communly yt stondyth [p. 35] of the whyte of the
eye and rownde abowte the tonycles and the blaknes of the eye.
And yt commyth with a grete furour and brynnyng and habundance of terys þat anoon the eyn bolne, and on such wyse þat
from þat tyme forth the pacyent may haue no reste nor slepe,

375 ffor euer yt semyth to hym þat hys eyn were ful of grauel or
thornes or smoke. To thys maner of sekenes, be yt yn yong
folkys or aged, thys ys the cure:

Take a sarcacollum album and bete yt wele to pouder yn a
brasym morter, and of pouder put the eye ful and lette hym ley
380 wyde opyn tyll the powder be consumed. And yn the [p. 36]
meanetyme make a plaster of flaxen herdys and wesshe þem
welle togydder yn cold water and presse out all the water yn
thyn honde. And then ley yt on the seke ey, the pacyent lyyng
alwey wyde opyn. And anoon thow schalt see þat he schal
385 begynne to rest and to sclepe.

Thys maner of infirmyte the grete lechys of Salerne clepyd
obtalmyam, but I, quod Benuonucius, calle yt torturam tenebrosam, ffor so much as it commyth with so greet a torment þat
it makyth the eye dymme and derke. And the forseyd medycyne
390 ys callyd pul[p. 37]uerem benedictum, the blessyd powder; ffor
with þat powder, wythoute ony oþer blode lettyng or purgacion
or oynement, I haue holpyn many of thys maner of sekenes.

Knowe ȝe þat euyl curyng, euyl kepyng, vnknowyng lechys,
folowyng errors for lak of dewe crafte with theyr impertynent
395 medycynes, add yn sorow vpon sorow and peyn opon peyne, by
occasyon wherof many a pacyent comme neuer to helth. And
yn sum occasyon of suche contraryous medycyns, the eyon with
all þeir concauytee apeeren wythout the lyddys, that þei be foul
disfygurde and [p. 38] dyshonurde and yit þei see not. And
400 when þei ar come to th<is> plyte, þere may no medycyne
helpe þem, forasmuche as the eye ys dyssauerd and departed
from hys inwarde syȝte or place and mortyfyed yn all hys substance. And yit sum oþer ther be þat by occasyon of obtalmie ar
gretly troublyde yn þere eyen, fumous and often wepyng for
405 evyll keepyng and for that they ete contraryous metys. But yit

400. this S] the H1

61

þei arn not vncurable. Wherfor yf ony such come to your cure, ffyrst pourge hys brayne with thies peletys:

Take polypodie, esule, myrabolanys, cytryne, [p. 39] rubarbe ana ounce 1; masticys, cubibys, saferon, spygnarde, nucys Indicem, cynamon ana a drame. And þan medyll them with mylke and yeue to the seke after hys strength. And after thys purgacion, yeue hym morne and yeue of the electuarie dyolibanum or Salernitanum, os yt ys sayd beforn in the cure of the iij curable cateract. And on the morn put yn hys ey of the powder callyd puluis nabetys (the makyng therof and the vertu yt schal be tauȝt hereafter yn the cure of the iij pannycles). And at eve put theryn of the powder callyde [p. 40] puluis Alexandrini, as it ys seyd a lytle before. And thys do tyll the pacyent be ful hoole, and yn meanetyme kepe hym from contraryus metys.

Now after the obtalmie I wyll speke of pannyclys and her curys, whych be gendryde of superhabundance of blode (as obtalmies be in dyuerse wyse). In tyme of euyl keepyng and after by grete peyne fallyng yn the heede ys causyd the mygreym, wherthrugh the peyne descendyth ynto the templys and ynto the [p. 41] browys and makyth the veynes to bete, of whych peynful betyng the eyon arn trowblyd. The pannyclys arn gendryd yn the eyon yn iiij wyse, as thus:

The fyrste pannycle apperyth yn the ey as the seyd of a corne clepyd in Laten milys and yn Ynglych myleseed. Thyes greynes or cornellys of myle growen yn the tonycle saluatrice; and in sum place they arn clepyd guttatici, and yn oþer places pedacelle, and in Naples þei ar callyd creature. The secunde pannycle ys that whych apperyth [p. 42] on the tonycle saluatryce lyke a spotte yn the face or lyk a frakyn or the scale of a fysch. The iijd apperyth on that on partye of the ey as a flake of snowe when yt snewyth. The iiijth ys when all the ey aperyth white and no blaknes aperyth neþer on the tonycle nor on the lyȝte.

The cure of the fyrst ys: put no medycyne nor withyn nor

62

440 wythoute, ffor þis infirmytee may not be curyd wyth laxatyvs
nor wyth pouders nor wyth coleryes nor wyth electuaryes nor
wyth cauteryes, ffor all þies raþer noye þan helpe. Ffor thys
maner [p. 43] of pannycle ys curyd wyth thys precious oynement:

445 Take xl tender croppys of bremell and stampe hem as smale
as sause; and a goode handful of rewe and powder of alabastre
halfe a pownde; fenkyl seed poudered halfe an vnce; oyle of
roses a pounde. All thyes encorporate togydder, put þem yn a
new erthen pott wyth a quarte of whyte wyne, and to all thyes

450 put iiij vnces of drye floures of camamyl and of wexe an vnce.
Then boyle yt wyth easy fyre tyll all the wyne be consumed and
wasted so ferforth that yt semeth to frye. [p. 44] After thys anon
put þerto the whyte of vj eggys and alway stere tyll þei be
yncorporate togydder; thanne streyne yt þorugh a lynnyn

455 cloyth. And thys oynement ys callyd preciosum vnguentum
alabastri, the prescyous oynement of alabaster. Wyth thys
anoynt the temples of the pacyent and the forhede down to the
browys, which oonly curyth thys pannycle þat aperyth as greynes of milie. Thys precyous oynement hath many grete vertues,

460 for not oonly yt avaylyth for thys manner of pannycle þat
apperyth as grene of milie, but also [p. 45]where any man fele
any dysease yn the body, lete hym anoynte hym þereof and he
schal fynde ease. And yf a man haue a wounde, let hym ley of
thys onement þertoo and yt schal clense yt and close yt. Also for

465 the toothake anoynte thy cheke þer ayenst, and anon yt slakyth
the payne. Also yf women haue payn yn ther matrice, ete of
thys oynement as a lectuarye and anoon schal be delyuerd of
ther payn. Also men in axesse ymade to be anoynted on the
stomake on the hondys and on the feete and the reynes, and

470 anoon to be dely[p. 46]uerd and releuyd. Also thys oynyment
ys for euery mygryme and for euery payne of the ey, yf the
pacyent be anoynted therwyth—the forhede, the templys, and
browys.

63

The secund panycle I wyll ȝe knowe. But yf yt be curyd anon
475   yn the begynnyng of the growyng þereof, yt wyll not be curyd
after (the pacyent schal wele se). Ffor when yt ys incarnate and
hardened vpon the tonycle, þow ȝe wolde wyth your twycchys
lyft it vp and kut yt wyth a rasoure, ȝe mowe not so sotyllye kut
yt but þat ȝe shuld kut the tonycle therwyth, wyth whych [p. 47]
480   kut all the substance of the ey shuld be destroyed anoon. Wherfore I counsel yow that when ȝe se thys maner of pannycle not
new but incarnate and harded vpon the tonycle of the eye, take
yt not in cure, for ȝe may haue no worschype þerof but hurtyng
your name and fame among the people. Neuerthelesse yf ȝe
485   comme þerto while yt ys new growe and not incarnate vpon the
saluatryce, cure yt on thys wyse:

Ffyrst yn the [the] begynnyng make a cauterye in the templys
wyth a rownde cautarye, whych as I schal shew you [p. 48]
afterwarde among my cautaryes, for fire drawyth and disso-
490   luyth and cons < umeth > and suffryth no pannycle to be incarnate vpon the tonycle. And so by drawyng dissoluyng and consumyng by þat place cauteryzed, thys maner of pannycle ys
consumyd wasted and dystroyed and the ey able to be claryfyed
with the medycyns folowyng. When thys cauterye ys made lyke
495   as seyd, anoon put into the pacyent ey, lying wyde open, of the
powder callyd puluus nabetus, whych [p. 49] schal be tauȝt
after. And whyle < he > lyeth wyth the powder yn hys ey, take
iiij crabbys and rost þem, doo awey the pyllys wythoute and the
coore wythyn, and incorporate them wyth the whyte of an egg
500   in maner of a oynement. And ley yt on a plaster of clene flexen
herdys and bynde yt to the eye wyth a lynnen cloyth. And so let
yt be from morn tyll yeue, and þen make a new plaster from
yeue tyl the morn. And thus shall ȝe cure al maner of pannycles

490. consumeth S] conseruyth H1
497. he S] omit H1

whyle they ar new, and the pacyent schall recouer lyȝt and syght

505   perfyȝtly, to the louyng of gode.

< *[f. 13] Of the therd pannicle and the cure of it*

< *Of the thridde maner of pannicle ys that the whiche apperethe fro the*
on partye of the eyȝe as it were whan it snowyth a fleke of snowe. And we
sayne that same cure ye shull do as we haue saide in the 2e pannicle, as ye

510   *haue afore, þat is to saye with a* < *ca* > *uterye in the templis and ye shull*
putte in the eyȝe of the pouder nabatis. But natheles putte therto with hym
this medicyn, the whiche also is gode ayenst the whitenesse of the eyȝen,
forwhi it blakethe the tonicle and it distroiethe the spotte and the white-
nesse, that is webbes, of the eyȝen, and this is the medicyne:

515   < *Take ounces 9 of fyne tree of gode aloes, and also hauethe a newe*
platter of stonye erthe full of firy colys. Than lay that aloes tree on the quyk
colys, and on that other side haue ye a moche clene basyn that maye
ouerkeuery þat stonen plater withe the colys, so that it may take all that
smoke and reseyue it into the basyn. And [f. 13v] that fume yreseyued,

520   *than haue ye a nabiatis ounces 9, poudred, and in that bacyn where that*
the fume of aloes ys receyued, medle hym theryn [hym theryn] with a
brasyn pestell till it be made into a right sotill pouder. With that forsaide
fume of the poudre, medle hem well togiders. Whan this poudre ys ymade
þus as y haue asayde, than do of this poudre twyes a day naturall, that is

525   *at the morwe and at euen, into the eyȝe. And aboue that laye a plastre*
ymade of applis, as I haue taught you in the secunde pannicle, þan bynde it
to withe a bonde till it come to his hele ayen. And we haue delyuered and
ycured many folke with these cures witheouten numbre.

< *Nowe we shull teche you of what spice ye shull make poudre nabatis*

530   *of, whiche is the properte to deliuer the secunde and the iijde pannicle. The*
zu < *c* > *ere nabatis ys made after Arabie tung and Saracenys speche, and*
Turkes clepen it zucre gylop. We Cristin men clepen it zucre nabatis and
also zucre candi of Alexandri. Of these zucre candi of Alisaunder we make

---

505. S adds the following: "Here my author left of to speake any further of the other 2
panicles. And beginneth to speake of the other infirmityes caused of flegme"
510. cauterye] tuterye H2
531. zucere] zuere H2

535

poudre nabatis, the whiche poudre doithe many grete merueiles to the pannicles [f. 14] of the ey3en. Ffirst it makethe nesshe that pannicle for his grete moystenes. Secunde it swagethe the ache for his swetenes and his mekenes. 3e it distroiethe redenes of ey3en for his purite of < h > is hete. 4e it fretethe the webbes in the ey3en for < h > is hardenes, forwhi or that it be dissolued and it be ybrought into water, myghtly it fretethe the webbe. 5 it

540

comfor< te > the the sight; for yeff any hete be in the ey3en it purifiethe it, and also it cler⌀ the sight and it quickethe the visible spirit. 6 fore [for] it constraynethe teres yef the teres were of colde humours, for thorugh his hete it withtemperethe the coldenes of humours.

< Of the 4⌀e pannicle and the cure of it

545

< Of the ferthe pannicle ys whan the ey3e apperethe all white and none blake ys ther yseyn, ney⌀er nothinge of the tonicle of the ey3en neither of the sight. Than wete the well that ⌀at fallethe fore the moche akthe that is comen doun by the mydward of the heuyd with grete wodenes and furosite, and it enclosethe the ey3en all aboute. And for that grete anguisshe of ak⌀e

550

the ey3e wexethe white and apperethe in colour as shynyng alabaustre, and the pacient fro ⌀ens [f. 14v] forward seethe nought or yif any of lyght shewe yit he seethe but feblyche. Ffor hym semethe that all the worlde ys white, and he may not knowe ne shewe o thing from anothir thinge, and his ey3en ben alway wateryng and all the naturall white of ⌀e ey3en appereth rede all

555

aboute the tonicle ywhited.

< The cure of this ys first ye shull make a cautarye in the neysshe of the heued, as ye shull see in our cauterijs. And whan ye haue ymade a cautery, take to whites of eyren and putte hem in a disshe that is newe and swynge hem till they make skume, and afterward lete it rest. And after that kest

560

away that skume; and that clere water putte theryn a pece of clene coton and, the ey3en yshitte, lay ther abouen x tymes in the daye and x sithes in the nyght till the pacient be parfitely hole. With this cures we haue ycured to the ffulle the 4e pannicle, fforwhy it is yprouyd and parfitelich it

537. his] is H2
538. his] is H2
540. comfortethe] comforthe H2

66

worshippithe the leches crafte. Wherefore bethe well ware in these foure
565 *pannicles and beth nought bolde to putte other medicynes into the eyʒe but*
thoo that we han wreten to you. Ffor I do you to vndirstonde þat these
pannicles were neuer withe none other [f. 15] medecyns that ben violent,
but rather they < engender > sorowe and woo and akthe more on anoþer
woo. >

570 [p. 50] Off the infyrmitees of flewme

And lyke as blode arne gendryd obtalmyes and pannycles,
ryʒte so by occasyon of flewme arn gendrid oþer dyuerse
sekenes. And specyally iiij, of whych the fyrst ys habundance of
terys by whos grete fluxe the eylyddys arn so molifyed and
575 made soft þat withyn grow herys whych pryk the balle of the ey
contynuelly. Of whych prykkyng the eyon be so troubled þat the
pacyent may not opon hys eyon. Som boystious and vnconnyng
leches pullen awey [p. 51] the herys, and þan pacyent seeth for a
tyme. But when the herys growe ayen, than commyth they to
580 wors astate, for the more þat þei be pullyd, the gretter and the
harder they waxen < and cause farr more greatter paine > –
and sum tyme for oon growyth iij or iiij. And tho pryk the eyon
as swynes brystyll and trouble so the eyon that the pacyent may
not vpon hys eyon, and many lesen her syght wyth all the
585 substance of þer eyon by occasyon of such heyres. Wherfore þis
dyssease must be cured oþerwyse þan thus.

Take ij nedylles of the len[p. 52]gth of thy lytyll fynger, and
put a threde thorugh the eyon of boyth, and bynde þem wele
togydder. Than with thy fyngers lyfte vp the ower eylyde, and
590 with these nedyllys take so of the ledder where theys herys
growe þat the pacyent may opon and schyt hys eyon. And þan
bynde wele thyse nedlys togydder at boyth endys, and so lett it
be tyl the nedyls fall away by þemselfe wyth the pese of ledder
that was betweyne þem. The whych doon, put no medycyne yn

568. engender] egreggyn H2
581. and cause . . . paine S] omit H1

595 the wonde þat the nedlys haue mayd, for yt shall hele wele
ynowe [p. 53] by ytselfe, but yf any pannycle or rankyll be
gendyrde on the ey by vyolence of the peyn and þat schall be
curyd with the powder callyd puluis nabetus put yn the ey twyes
on the day tyl the ey be claryfyed and ful helyd. And wyth thys
600 sekenes of eyon, quod my autor, I founde moo ywoxen yn
Calabur þen in ony oþer prouynce, and specyally of women.
And thys preciosus powder we calle puluis nabetus, and yt ys
mayd of sugyr, whych in Arabyk tong the Sarasyns call sugar
gelypp, and Crysten men cal yt sugar candy of Alex[p.
605 54]ander. Thys powder ys goode and syker to hole al sekenes of
eyon.

The second sekenes cawsyd of flewme in the eyon ys when þei
appere trobled and ful of venys closed with a pannycle so that
the pacyent may not wele se. And thys sekenes we calle pannum
610 vitreum off whych thys ys the [the] cure:

Ffyrst at the begynnyng doo shaue of all the hede, and than
cauterye hym with a rownde cauterye yn the soft of hys hede
and wyth a long cauterye yn hys templys. Whych so doon, put
yn hys eyon oonys of þis pouder of candye onys of the daye [p.
615 55] tyl he receyue ayen ful syȝte. And twyes yn the monyth
pourge hym wythoute wyth pelettes callyd pulule Iherosolomitane, and when he goyth to bede lete hym resceyue of our
electuarye clepyd dyaolibanum Salernitanum tyl he be hole.
And of thys sekenes we founde many mo pacyentes yn Tuscia
620 < and > Marchia þen yn ony oþer contreys.

The thyrde infirmytee caused of flewme: when the ey
apperyth carnous or fleshly, whych carnosyte or fleshelynes, yf
yt be woxen harde vpon the eye a yere or ij or mo, yt may not
be cured, neiþer wyth [p. 56] [wyth] pouders, neþer coloryus,
625 for it shuld nothyng avayle. Wherfore, as I sayd before, the
pacyentes hede must be shauyn and cauteryzede ffyrst, as I

620. and] omit H1

sayd yn the cure before. And on the nexte day after, opyn the
pacyentes eyon wyth your fyngurs and with a rasure cut all the
carnosytee, so warly and so sotylly þat ȝe touche not the tonycle
630   saluatrice, whych Iohannycius clepyth the coniunctyfe. But
rounde abowt the tonycle betwene the blak and the whyte, soft
and sotylly cut yt tyll ȝe haue reysed all the carnosytee. Whych
so doon, fyll the ey ful [p. 57] of the powder of candie without
ony oþer thyng. Then doo the pacyent shitt hys ey and þeron ley
635   a plaster of coton or of flaxen herdys wyth the whytte of an egg,
and xv days after chaunge the plaster twyes on a day. And after
xv days make thys plaster: take an[d] handful of an herbe callyd
cardus benedictus, sowthystyl yn Englych, stampe yt wele and
medyl yt with halfe the whyte of an egg. And make a plaster of
640   coton or flaxen herdys and ley yt on the ey iij days, remeuyng
the plaster euery [p. 58] daye, eche day twyes, morn and yeue.
And after iij dayes complete, leue all plasters and lete the
pacyent sye with open ey. And euery daye at morn put yn the
sore eyon of the powder callyd puluis benedictus, and at eue of
645   the powder callyde puluis nabetus, tyl he be perfyȝtly hoole.
And yn the meanetyme let hym abstene hym from elys,
oyneones, and befe and all oþer queysy metys. And with thys
maner of medycyne, quod myn autor, I haue holpen and curede
without nombre of people. Of thys sekenes, quod he, I fonde
650   mo in Sardo[p. 59]nia than yn oþer countrees.

     The forth sekenes causyd of flewme yn the ey is when the
eyon apere bolleyn and be allweys wepyng, and the pacyent
may not opyn hys eyon for the ponderosyte and the heuynes of
the ouerlyddys. And yf ȝe wyll, quod he, be verryly certyfyed of
655   thys sekenes, turne the ouerlydde of the ey with your fyngers
and ȝe schal se it appere all fatty, and the fatnes shall be greynous as much as the greynes of a myle. Whych sekenes Sarasyns
and yn Arabye ys callyd iherafrumaxyn, þat ys to sey scab yn
the eye. [p. 60] And thys sekenes ys gendred of superhabun-
660   dance of salt flewme. To whych sekenes do thys cure:

69

Fyrst ȝe must pourge the stomake and the brayne of the
pacyent with þis resceyte: Take turbyt, aloes, epatyk, rubarbe
lyche of ycche an vnce; then take the juce of the roote of
walworte a pounde and the forseyd thynges poudered and reso-
665   luyd yn the sayd jus. And let yt stond all a nyght, and betyme or
the morn clense yt, and lete the pacyent take þerof fastyng a
good quantite. And on the nexte day after that wyth your
fyngurs tornyth the eylyddys, and [p. 61] softly with a twycche
lyft the carnositee and with a rasure begynne to cut the greynes
670   yn fatnese tha<t> ys vnder the eyelede, euyn from that oon
lacrymal to the tooþer. Whych doon, plaster the eye wyth herdys and the whytte of an egg, and so do ix days, eche daye
chaungyng the plaster twyes. And after the ix days lay þerto the
playster gracious aforseyd, <[f. 18] *the whiche ys ymade of cardus*
675   *benedictus with the white of an eye*>, twyes on the daye iij days
foloyng, after whych tyme lat the pacyent haue hys eyon opyn.
And alwey at yeven put yn hys ey of oure colerye callyd colerium Alexandrinum, whych ys tauȝt before yn [p. 62] the cure
of the thyrde pannycle, tyl he be perfytely hoole. And wyth
680   thys, quod he, I haue curyd muche people.

And of thys sekenes [sekenes] I founde moyste yn Barbarye
among the Sarasyns. And when I was þer, quod he, I fonde
women vsyng thys cure: They tooke the braunches of the fyg
tree and turnyd the eyelyddys, and with the leuys they rubbyd
685   the sore place tyl the eyledys weren all blodye. And many were
amendyd þerby, but yt lastyd not long. And som rubbyd þat
fatnes wyth suger; for a tyme þei were amendyd, but soon [p.
63] after yt tornyd ayen into the fyrste estate.

And now I wyl teche yow practysers a merveilous and a
690   precious lectuarye for the forsayd terys, and yt ys thys: Take
olibam, castorij, nootmygges, nucys Indie, clouys, cubibes ana
an vnce; and of the leuys of laurei, spynarde, saferon, cardo-

670. that] tha H1

momi ana a quartron; halfe an vnce seedys of dylle; of smalache, basylycon seede, of alexander, of annes, and of fenel ana
695   halfe an vnce; drye neppe, pulyal, ysop, sede of rewe ana iiij
drammes; seed of henbane, whytte popee, muske, [p. 64] campher ana a dram. Bete all thyes to powder and sotylly sarce
them, saue the olybanum; that must be boylyde wyth claryfyed
hony tyl yt be molton. Then take yt from the fyre and power yt
700   ynto a feir plater large and of tree wyth the oþer powders, and
wyth a lytyl ladyl styre yt togyddyr tyll the spycys be yncorporate wyth the hony; and lete yt be kept styll yn the same
plater. And ȝe shall cure your pacyentes: Yeue them at yeue
when þei goo to bede of thys lectuarye the quantite of a ches-
705   teyne. And thys lectuarye, quod he, ys callyd meruelous [p. 65]
and prescious ffor yt doth many prescious merueleus. Hyt dystroyth the teres and flewme, yt warmyth the brayn, it puttyth
awey the peyne of the mygreyme, it openyth the eyon, it
releuyth the eylyddys and clarifyth the syght. It is also good for
710   the eyon þat haue the gowte and the palsye, item for them þat
haue loost their speche or haue impedyment yn spekyng. Al
thyes I haue preuyd, quod he, and as I here wryte so haue I
founde and manny haue I holpen.

Off the infirmytees causyd of coolore [p. 66]

715   Now after thys, quod the autor, I shall trete of the sekenes of
the eyon causyd of coler, whych byth ij. Wherof the first ys
causyd of superhabundance of coler yn the stomake, of the
whych ys resoluyd a corrupte fumosytie þat ascendyth vp to the
brayn with greete furowre and pyne, wherof the eyon be so
720   troublyd þat betwene þem and their obiecte, þat ys the thyng, ys
yn the maner of a shadowe or a clowde. And yit the eyon appere
feire and bryght, and neiþer yn the eyon nor wythoute ys no
spot [p. 67] aperyng; and þerfore the defaute of thys ys not yn
the eye but in the stomake, and þerfore no medycyne schal be
725   put yn the ey but in the stomake. And the cure þerof shal be
with a electuarye mytigatyf and aperytyf, whych shal swage the

peyne and opyne the opylate holes — neruys — þat þe uisible spyryt maye frely passe þereby. And þus shal be the lectuarye
made:

730   Take rubarbe, esule minorys, rede sawnders, mirabolys
cytrine ana iiij vnces; the rotys of fenel, sperages, bruscies, parcely, smalach, < u > i < t > acelle, cycorye, [p. 68] capyllys
veneris ana of eche an handful; polypody of the oke ij vnces.
Boyl all thies herbys yn feir water to the halfe be wasted, and

735   þen clense yt. Than take the forseyd spycys wele powderd and
put þem to the seyd lycour wyth ij pounde of suger and make
þerof a syrup laxatyff. But when ȝe put the spycys and suger,
beware þat yt boylle not after but lytle, for þan shal the spycys
lese theyr wertu and her myght. And when it ys redy clense yt

740   ageyn, and of thys syrup lete the pacyent drynk twyes yn the
weke. [p. 69] And yn the menetyme lete hym abstene hym from
contraryous metys and from such as byth of harde dygestyon,
and also lete hym be cauteryzed on the templys besydys the erys
as ȝe, quod he, schall se assygned in my cauteryes.

745   The secunde sekenes causyd of color ys whan þer aperyth
vpon the tonycle of the eye before the syght as yt were a thyn
clowde yn a clere eyre, and vnneth yt may be seyn. And thys
sekenesse fallyth not but to þem to whom and yn whom coler
reygnyth and when þei be yn an accesse. And when the acces ys

750   [p. 71] goon, thys dysease remayneth for lak of due cure
betyme. And for þat absteyne not from contraryous metys, but
for thys sekenes thys ys the cure:

    Take a saphyr and breke yt yn a morter ynto sotyl powder,
and the powder to be kept yn a vessyl of golde. And onys on the

755   day put of þat yn the pacyentes eye, and he shall be hoole yn
schort tyme. The same doth the galle of a bawson yf yt be dryed
and powderred and put yn the eye < [f. 20] *onys a day, and he*

732. uitacelle VP1, f. 251] sicacelle H1
750. H1 omits 70 from the page numbers, going from 69 to 71.

shall be deliuered at full thorugh this medicyne. Also take fenell sede ounces
iiij on the tother side and thre parties of poudre nabatis on the tone side,
760 *and in a brasyn morter make poudre of the forsaide gumme and medle it*
and afterwarde do hem bothe into the morter togiders till bothe be right
sotill and do this poudre into the eyȝe. And fforsothe it dothe thre thingis:
first it freteth the webbe, 2e and it softethe and clerethe the eyȝe and it
conseruethe light till <h> is lyues ende. Wherfor on þe [f. 20v] *gumme*
765 *of fenell Ypocras and Galien and all the olde leches were accorded togeders*
and helde it for a high medecyn, and wete ye well that they nemenyd it none
gumme but fenell, for þey nould naught shewe wherein his vertue was. And
for certayne we wole shewen ffor they praysed the herbe and the sede but
nought the gumme, though they couthe hit but they hidden where that the
770 *verray trewth was. Wherfor with that holy herbe we haue delyuerd many,*
and that þat was hidde nowe it is open and proued. >

Off the infyrmytees of malencolye [p. 72]

For the humor malencoly ys gendyrd y<n> myche peple,
many dyuerse dysease yn eyon come þerof, wherof oon ys thys.
775 Sumtyme for the habundance of malencolye the brayn ys so
troublyd þat the nerfe obtyk ys so opylate and stoppide þat the
vysyble spyryt may not passe the ryght wey. And when thys
nerfe ys oppylate and ouerleid þen aperen afore the pacyentes
eyon as yt were fleyng flyes yn the ayre on the daylyght. And of
780 a lanterne of lyȝte or of the moone, yt [p. 73] semyth þat yt were
iiij, and yf he loke yn the face of a man yt semyth to hym the
same. Thys maner of sekenes yt happenyth to them raþer þat be
naturally malycolyus when þei vexen aged, raþer than to men of
oþer complexion. Wherfor the practysers when ȝe se such a
785 pacyent put no medycyne yn hys eye but make hym a lectuarye
mytygatyff and aperytyff, whych schall swage the peyn and
open the opylacion of the hole neruys þat the spyryt of syght
may passe esely by them. And þus it shal be made: [p. 74]

764. his] is H2
773. yn] y H1

Take suger, lycoryse, eufrasie, siler mownten, and hylwort
790 ana halfe a pounde; off the seedys of rewe, basylycon, urtice
vltra marine, fenel, alexander, smalege, caruy ana ij vnces;
masticus, clowys, notmygges, cynomom, cubibe, gumme of
almandys, cerase, pyonie, gummarum Arabici, dra[ga]ganti,
safron halfe an vnce; grana cytemorum, pioniorum an vnce. All
795 thyes muste be betyn togydder to smal pouder and wele sarsed
and þan confect wyth goode suger and make a lectuarye. And of
thys lete the pacy[p. 75]ent ete fyrst at morn and laste at yeven,
and he shal be hoole. Thys sayd lectuarye ys not oonly good for
thys sekenes but also for all tho whych see not clerely but haue
800 yn maner a myste yn þer eyon, causyd eiþer of thouȝt and grete
heuynes of a grete weepyng or of wacche or of fastyng or of such
oþer. And þerfor thys lectuarye ys clepyd clarificacio oculorum,
this ys the clarifyers of eyon.

Ther ys also anoþer sekenes causyd of malyncolye and yt ys
805 when the payne sodonly ascendyth ynto [p. 76] the eyon and so
greuou<s>ly þat it semyth the eyon wolde stert oute of theyr
places, and þei aperyn passyngly bollen. And of thys maner of
pacyentes som lese holy þer syght, and som seen but feblye.
And not forthan all thyes may be holpe yf they be cured yn the
810 begynnyng of theyr sekenes wyth thyes medycynes that I shal
sey yow. Ffyrst the stomake and the brayn must be porged wyth
our pelates of comforth, whych ar made on thys wyse:

Take aloes, epatyk, mirabolys cytryne, tur[p. 77]byt, saunders, citrine, rubarbe ana half an vnce; scamony, safrone,
815 balsami, mirre, mastyci, lygnum aloes, olibanum album, agaricus, nuces Indie, succum <liqueritiae>, the seed of smalache,
letuce, cicorie, basylicon ana of each a drame. Bet all ynto
powder and confecte þem wyth the jows of roses and make
pelatys, and yif yt the pacyent after hys power. And when the

806. greuously] greuouly H1
816. liqueritiae S] siquericus H1

820 stomake and the brayn ben powrged, ley on the ey my plaster
clepyd emplastrum laudabile, whych ys made on thys wyse:

Take [p. 78] sowre apples, þat ys crabbes, and roost þem
hoote yn the embrys tyll they soft; then voyde away the parow
and the core and bruse þem wele yn a morter. And to iiij
825 crabbys put the whyte of an egg glayre and bray þem togeddyr
tyl þei be incorporatte yn maner of an oynement. And of thys
lawdable plaster ley on flexen herdys and plaster yt on [on] the
eye twyes on the daye, morn and yeuen. And yn thys wyse ye
shal cure thys maner of disease yf it be aplied and vsed at the
830 begynnyng. Of thys plaster thyes be vertues: [p. 79] ffyrst yt
swagyth the bolnyng, it settyth the eye fyxe yn hys place, it
lesseth the payn, and refreshyth the syght; and for thies causes I
cal it laudable, that ys worthy to be praysed.

Also superhabundance of the humor of malencolye is often
835 gendryd yn the ey a dysease callyd vngula, a nayle, for it ys
muche lyke a fyngernayle, and begynnyth comonly to growe in
lacrimabili minore, þat ys to sey yn the corner of the eye to the
ere-ward. And the course of the growyng ys toward the pupil,
þat ys to sey to the syȝte. And yf it [p. 80] be not cut away or it
840 ocupye the pupil and let the syȝght, afterwarde it wyll not be
easely curyd. Also sumtyme þere growyth anoþer vngyll in the
corner of the eye nexte the noose, and yf thies ij happyn to be
knyt togydder and to occupye all the eye and to let all the
syȝght, þan it ys more hard to cure. But not forthan boyth be
845 curable but by grete dyscrecion and sotyl workyng or wrythyng
of the honde, and þis must be the cure:

Take a twych of syluer and þerwyth sotylly lift vpe [p. 81] the
vngle from the tonycle <[f. 22v] *and so with a rasour kutte her*>,
procedyng forthe to the lacrymal where he toke hys growyng.
850 And when it is all cut awey wyth a rasour sotilly, lete the
pacyent spere yn hys eye and lay þerto a plaster of the whyte of
an egg x dayes folowyng, twyes on the day renewed, whych so
past lete hym wash hym with hote water. And þan put yn hys ey

at morn and euyn of my powder callyd puluis nabetus tyl the
855   eye be clere sufficyently. And yn the menetyme lete hym
absteyne hym from contraryous metys, and noon oþer medycyne yn the eye. [p.82]

It happyth sum tyme þat the malencolyous humor habundant
yn the brayn begynnyth to haue hys course by the eyon, and for
860   the superhabundance þereof it makyth the eyledys to wexe drye.
And þat drynes tornyth after to an ycche and to brynnyng, and
the cause of thys brynnyng and ycche ys for that he tooke no
purgacion yn the begynnyng of the sekenesse nor absteyned
from contraryous metys. Off thys dysease thus ys the cure: yf
865   the pacyent be yong, lete hym blode on the veyne yn the myddys of the forhede. Whych so doon [p. 83] cure hym with a
colerie clepid colerium ruborum, thus made:

Take xlti tendyr croppys of the bremyl and stampe them as
smale as sauce and put it yn a new erthen pot with a quarte of
870   goode whyte wyne and boyle it wyth an esy fyre tyl halfe be
consumede. Than clense yt and kepe it yn a glasse, wherof
twyes yn the day put yn the pacyentes eye and noon oþer thyng
tyl he be hole. And thys colerie ys goode ageyne al skaldyng and
rednesse of the maladie of the forseyd sekenes. Quod the autor,
875   I fonde mo yn Rome than yn any [p. 84] othir prouince.

Moreoure of such superfluyte of malencolie sumtyme þere
grouyth a corupte humor wythout the eye betwyxte the place
where the here growyth and the eyelydde, whych bolnyth not
oonly the eyelydde but all the eye wyth halfe the face, but it
880   hurtyth not the eye. And men of Tuskan calle it humeris benedictum; them of Rome call it nexionam; and men of Cicile and
Grekys cal it papulam; but the citramowntayns and Frenshe-
men and oþer cal it maledictam — and no wonder, for yt growyth with grette soroues and [p. 85] grete peyn. And thies ben
885   the knowyng þerof: it makyth the eyledys al harde, red, and
bolnyn and kepyth the ey so shyt þat the pacyent may not open
it. Off whych disease thys is the cure:

Take fyne pure flowre of olde whete and ȝelkys of egges as
much of ech an vnce; of safron a drame. And stampe them wele
890   togeddyr wyth womans mylke, mollifi yt tyl yt be as an oynement, wherof make a plaster and lay it to the sore. And
betweyne the ij eylyddys ley a smayl lyst of lynnen cloyth to
kepe [p. 86] [that on] þat noon of the plaster entre ynto the ey.
And iij tymes doo þis plaster. It gederyth toogheder all the
895   humors into oon place; than after rypeth it; and for the þryd yt
swagyth the payn. And wyth þis many haue ben holpen of thys
disease.

Anoþer medicyne also for the same: Take a lilie roote and
roost yt yn hoot embers; take also crabbys and rooste hem yn
900   the hoote fyre or embrys — is better tyll þei be roost. Þan avoyde
the perrowr and the core and stampe þem and the root [to]
togydder, as mych by weyght of the [p. 87] toon as of the tooþer,
tyl þei be welle incorporate and temper þem with the whitte of
egges tyll þei be wele liquyde. And plaster the sore wyth this
905   onyment tyl all the humor be consumyd and that the ey may
open and shytte. And on the stepe of the wonde there the sore
was ley on an oynement callyd vnguentum subtile, whych ys
made thus:

Take aloe, epatik, hennys grece, oyle of bitter almandys, and
910   white waxe ana of ycche one ounce, and incorporate them
togheder into an oynement. And þis shal consowdyn and subtilizen so the [p. 88] skyn of the wonde þat þer shal no step
apperyn yn the wonde.

Also I counsel yow þat ye haue wyth you vnguentum alabas-
915   trum, and yn euery cure of the eyon onys yn the day, þat is at
even, anoynte the pacyentes forhede, templys, and browis
þerwyth, ffor þat helpyth your medicyns and swagyth the peyne
and suffryth not the humors to descend to the hurt place and it
makyth the pacyent to haue rest.

920   Moreoure, quod Beneuucius, I wyl þat ȝe practysers

77

< know > that many of þem þat suffre this seid sekenes [to] cum
[p. 89] to me with þeir eylydys reuersed foule for lak of suffi-
cyent cure, as þei sey to me, and so yt was yn whos cure yt
procedid. Ffor wyth a rasor I deuyed it suttilly and discretely

925 the eylyd from the cycatryes of the wonde, so þat the eyelede
myght turne up and down. Which so doon, I made a lytyl
pylowe of lynnen cloth yn the maner of a lytyl chyldys fynger
and wett it in the whyte of an egg and layd þer vpon and bonde
it to wyth a lynnen bande to the nexte remeuyng aȝen. And so

930 contynue þis [p. 90] medycyne daylly to the xv daye, and than I
made an oynement of hennys grece and of whyte wexe. And
þerwyth I anoynted the pelowe lyke as I dyd before wyth the
whyte of an egg and leyd it on the cicatryce or on the wonde,
like as I haue doon before tyl it was perfiȝtly sensowdid and the

935 eylyde hole and yn good astate. Or els sumtyme I made a
pelowe of a sponge and leyd it on the wounde, for the propurte
of the sponge is to distroye waste flech, to drawe and to quyken
the spiryt [p. 91] of the blode, and to consowdyn and knit the
wounde and to bryng yt to good astate.

940 And on thys wyse, quod he, I cured all that hade þere eylydys
turnyd by the same cause. Neþerthelees of thys turnyng of the
eyleddis of superhabundance of superfluite of blode not curid
wythyn a yere, beware the practisers that ȝe enter not the vtter
parte of the eyelydde, but wyth a twycche sotilly lifte vp the

945 corner where the wast fleche ys vnder the eyelyd. And wyth a
rasur cutt it so discretly þat ȝe touche not the parte of the eylede
that [p. 92] the here growyth. Whych so doon, ley þerto such
smale pelatis as it ys saidyn the cure before, and change it twyes
on the day till it be ful hoole. And of thys maner of seke folkys I

950 found moyst yn Tuskeyn than yn any oþer prouince.

And also of the malencolyus humor, quod the autor, ther is
gendrid yn many men a sekenes that growyth betwene the nose

921. know S] omit H1

78

and the ey, and it apperyth lyke the pece of a long and it < is >
grauelous and voydyth allway fylth, and communly it towchyth

955 withyn the ouer eyelede and also the neþer. And [p. 93] in many
placis thys sore is clepyd muri or wulgalpus, off whych thys ys
the cure:

Wyth a twych sotylly lyft vp the sore and wyth the poynt of a
rasour cut yt vp by the roote. And then wyth a hoote yron

960 cauteryse it yn the place where the sore tooke hys orygynal
begynnyng so weryly that ȝe hurt not the eye, and annoynt it
with the oynement callyd vnguentum subtile tyll it be hoole.

In the fyrst partye of thys tretys, ȝe practysers, quod my
autor, I declared to yow [p. 94] what an eye is and how it ys

965 maid, after myn opynyon and oþer menys also, and what is a
cateracte and how many spycys be þereof curable and how
many vncurable, and how the cure of the curable ys and how þe
cure of the vncurable ys by an easy delyuerance of honde by a
craft callyd ars acuaria, that is the crafte of the nedyl. And after

970 yn the secunde partye I tauȝt yow of the infirmitees of eyon that
be caused inwarde by occasyon of distemperance of the iiij
humors, þat [p. 95] ys to wyt blode, color, flewme, and malyncolye, and þeir cures. And now yn thys thyrde partye and last of
my tretys, I wyll tel yow of þies hurtis and diseases causyd yn

975 eyon from wythouteward, as wyth smytyng of stekkys and
stonys and staues or ony such oþer. Wherfore here ere that I
procede to any specyall cure, I generally counseyl yow that
when ȝe se any suche come to yow, socowre them wyth the
whyte of an egg — and as sone as ȝe mowe, leyng to the ey a

980 plaster made of flexen hurdys and the whyte of [p. 96] an egg.
And yff it happen for the grete payn the humurs of the eye be
distroyd and dyssoluyd, and thys plaster renewith iiij sythes on
the day and twys on the nyȝte xv days togydder. And yf it
happyn by the hurte takyn the tonycle to be hurte or brokyn,

953. is S] omit H1

985 put twyes on the day and oonys of the nyght of a medycyne
founde be practyffe callyd virtus a deo data, whos makyng shal
be tauȝt anoon after. But [not] forþan ley not the forseyd plaster
tyl the forseyd tyme be past, and also foryetyth not anoyntyng
the pacyentys templys, hys forhede [p. 97] and his browes with
990 the prescyous oynement of alabastrum. And yf þei that be hurte
or smyten wyth thys be not curyd on the seid wyse betymes at
the begynnyng ere that theey begynne to bolne or to roote, þei
shal neuer be cured nor helyd wyth any oþer medycyne.

 Ffor I wyll ȝe knowe iij grete vertuous of the white of an egg,
995 and specyally for suche smytyng. The first it swagith the sorow
and the payn, the secunde it constrenyth the humors of the eyon
and purifyeth the eyon, the thyrd it suffryth no superfluyte of
humors [p. 98] to come into the eyon. And as for the medycyne
callyd virtus a deo data that knyttyth and sowdeth the tonycle
1000 ageyn yf it be brokyn, and it is made on thys wyse:

 Take xij strenus of new freshe leyd egges of white hennys and
put them in a morter and labur them wele with a pestel tyl thei
be wele yncorporate togydder yn maner of a oynement. And
þan put it yn a vessel of glase and put it yn the eye, as it ys seyd
1005 before, twyes on the daye and oonys on the nyght. Ffor lyke as
othyr consolydatyfe oynementys [p. 99] consowdyn and purifye
othir wondys, so thys vertu youen of god consowdyth the tonycle of the eye yf it be hurte and purifie < th > the eye. And with
thys ryght vertuous medycyne many one haue I cured and
1010 holpen — men, women, and chyldren — yn dyuers placys.

 Amonge whych yn a cetee callyd Messana was brought to me
a chylde whos eye was oute yn the myddys so that I myght se iij
humers, and wyth thys forseyde medycyne I saued hys eye
hoole. But he myght not see for hys ey was cataracte of the
1015 vyolence of the [p. 100] stroke, as it ys declaryd beforn yn the
fyrst spice of the curable cataract. Wherfore I lete hym be so iiij

1008. purifieth] purified H1

80

monethys after tyll the cataract was confermed, and þan I cured hym as I haue tauȝt beforn yn the curable cataract. On thys wyse shall ȝe cure all tho þat arn hurte in the ey wyth stroke or

1020 smytyng—and not os lewde leches arn wont to doo wyth a plaster made of waxe and powder of comyn, whych they leyd hoot to the ey hurte and broken. For yf the tonycle of the eye be hurte or brokyn, anoon it draw[p. 101]yth all the substance of the eye and consumyt the humors. For wex of his propurtee

1025 drawyth and consumyth, and commyn dyssoluyth and meltyth. And thus by drawyng, dyssoluyng, and consumyng, the eye ys distroyed and ys foule dysfigured. And the ey be smytyn and hurte wythoute brekyng of the tonycle, than this plaster drawyth þereto the spyrit and the humors and causyth grete sorowe

1030 rounde abowte the eye, and so betyth boyth the ey and the templys that often the ey ys wasted and dystroyed þerby, as I haue often [p. 102] founde yn dyuers placys. Also sum haue lost þeir syȝte wyth plasters made of wormewode and olibanum and of such hote and dissouatyfe thyng. Wherfore I counsel you to

1035 beware of all suche plasters, and haue allweye yn all hurtys of eyon caused of owtwardys by stroke or smytyng to the gracyous medycyne of the whyte of egges that I haue tolde, yf ȝe wyll not erre.

But here it ys to be noted and vnderstonde that yn my Laten

1040 <co>py lacked an hoole chapytere, in which tretys of [p. 103] hurtys taken aboute the eyon, as by strokys of the forehede and the browys, the eylyddes, the boyth lacrymalles, the temples, and such oþer of their cures. And moreouere the nexte chapyter folowyng in the begynnyng lakked sumwhat, but not muche as

1045 I suppose, wher he tretyth of watry eyon and of teres, of corrupte humors lyke teres whych leches callen festeles.

<[f. 28v] *Of smytyng of* [f. 29] *þe eyȝeliddes and in the temples and þe lacrimal place and þe cure þerof*

1040. copy] apy H1

< *Now we shull teche of the smytyng the whiche ben ayenst the eyʒe, as*
1050   *in the eyʒeliddis and in the templis and of the lasse lacrimale place and in*
bone that is vndre the nether eyʒelid. And we say yif a man be ysmete in the
eyʒeliddes and that smytyng be moche, and it towche þe bone that is
abought the eyʒe though it towch not the eyʒe; the eyʒe apperethe clere and
neuerthelesse hit hathe losten his lyght, ffor that smytyng neruus opticus is
1055   *stoppid in so moche that the visible spirite may nought come to the eyʒe.*
Also þe smytyng of the templis, it distourblethe the humours of the eyʒen;
fforwhy the pacient may nought clerelich se summe tyme, and yef it so be it
is vndre the eyʒelid in the nether partie so that it towchethe the bone that is
vndre nether eyʒelid—also he seythe nought though he haue a clere eyʒe.
1060   *Wherfor whan ye see any such, beholdethe into þat eyʒe and yef the balle of*
the eyʒe be brode or yif it be more than his felawe, knowe ye well that he
seithe nought. And yif the pacient sey that he seith, loke yif the appill of the
eyʒe yef it is [f. 29v] *made brode and constreyned it is to leue that he seiþ,*
forwhy the visible spirit comyng by the holwe synewe to his oute passage
1065   *makethe the eyʒe appill to wexe abrode and to constrayne. And yef it be*
nought ygone abrode and to constrayne, as it doþe in an hole eyʒe, and
though me semeth that he haue a clere eyʒe as the tother eyʒe [eyʒe] is clere;
whan he hathe these signes, as we haue ysaide, dothe no cure ffor the
holowe nerffe is so stoppid that the visible spirite by none wey may nowght
1070   *come to the eyʒe. And knowithe well that the senewe holwe most is stopped*
in hem that ben ysmete all aboute the eyʒe than in other causes, as it farethe
with men þat vsen swevyng and ben ypleased with suche doing labour or
betyngges or for fastyng or for teres or for melancolye humours and suche
othir doynges.
1075   < *Of smytyng in þe forheued atwix the browes or on þe nose side and þe*
cure þerof
     < *Smete in the forhede atwene the two browez and the nose on the to*
side (or on that other side, and it fallethe otherwhile), ther wexethe a
maner of corrupte humour goyng oute by the poyntes of the eyʒeliddes
1080   *biside the nose, as it were teres. And leches clepen þat humour fistule for*
it wexethe as it were rothed ymeynte with teres, and his cours allwey it
habundeþ [f. 30] *and wexethe more and more and it entrethe into the*

eyȝen and than they appere alwey teryfull. > Wherfore, quod
Benuynucius, of them oure lorde Ihesu yaue knowlege and
1085   experiens of the infirmytees of eyon, humors and complex-
yons, and the cures. Yf practysers wyll [p. 104] verely be
certyfyed wheþer the humor be a ffistula or a clere tere, do
þus: puttyth your secunde fyngers ende, whych ys callyd index
(the shewyng fynger), betwene the nose and the lacrimall,
1090   besyde the neþer eyelede, and þere shall ȝe se the corrupte
humor that is the mater of the fystyl goyng oute by the poyntys
of the eyeleddys betwene the nose and the eye. But many
boystus leches and ignorant, not knowyng the very place of
yssuyng of the corrupte, whych ys the mater of the fystyll, but
1095   weenyng that the goyng out of the corrupcioun were yn the [p.
105] myddys of the lacrymal besydys the nose betwyxt boyth
the eyeledys, and þei vsen for to cure a craft that ys a cause of
lesyng of manny mans syȝthtys. And it ys thus:
        They taken an hoote yron and make a cauterye vpon the nose
1100   yn the myddys of the lacrimall betwyx the ouere ylede and the
neþer lyd, weenyng for to dry vp the place where the corrupt
mater of the fystyl ys gendryd. But þei do not curee but deforme
foule the face yn the place whych þei cauteryze, and many, as I
haue seyd, deforrem and dystreyen the syȝth [p. 106] of the
1105   vysyble synews that arn clepyd nerui optici, goyng betwyxt
besyde the nose, by the cautaryzacion ben dried and the syȝte
destroyed. Wherfore yf ȝe wyll not dysteyne your name nor hurt
your pacyentes in cure of thys maner of fystyl, leue thys forseyd
lewde craft and do as I schall teche yow:
1110   Ffyrst clense the pacyentys stomake wyth the peletys of Ierusalem wherof the makyng ys tauȝt before. Whych purgacion
made, þen ȝe shall make a lytle insysyon wyth the poynt of a
rasor betwyxt the neþer eylyd and the nose, so dyscre[p. 107]tly
that ȝe touch not the eyelede and the nose neþer the substance of
1115   the eye. And thys incysion or kuttyng shal be but oonly þorugh
the skyn in lenghtwyse. In whych yncysion put the grane of a

fecche and lay þeron a lytle pylowe made of lynnen cloth and bynd it wyth a lynnen bende that the fecche remoue not from the place where it is leyd, and so lete it lye tyl the nexte day.

1120 Than remoue the fecche and yn the hole that it hath made ley of the coresey and mortyificat powder whych I shall teche yn the ende of the tretis [p. 108] ageyne all maner of fystylles whersoeuere they be. Whych powder put yn, do the pacyens shyt hys eye that the powder may not entre, or vpon the eyelyd lay a

1125 plaster of coton or flexen hardys iwet yn the whyte of an egg, and bynd it þerto wyth a lynnen bande tyl the nexte day. And þan anoynte yt or ley þerto clene freshe swynes grece tyl the mortifyed fleshe be reysed vp wyth the powder and the place remayne opyn. And than shal ȝe se the place putrifyed wher the

1130 begynnyng of the corrupte mater of the fystyl was and how the cowrs [p. 109] þereof yn the lacrymall shal be dryed. And after thys take a lytle pece of a sponge the quantyte of a fecche and ley yt yn the hoole that the powder mayd tyl it be pourgyd and dryed, ffor the propurte of the spounge ys to opyn, to consume

1135 wykkyd humors. And when the place ys dryed boyth be the poynt of the lacrymall and the cicatryce made by the fyrst incysyon, than leue the sponge and ley þereto nat els but fayre lynet of feyr lynnen cloth wythoute ony maner of oynyment tyl yt be perfyȝtly consowded — and so shall the <y> be delyuerd

1140 wythout perell. [p. 110] Neuerthelees euery nyȝte whyle he ys yn curyng when he goth to bedde, yeue hym of oure electuarie, callyd electuarium mirabile, the quantite of a chasteyn.

Now I haue shewed, quod he, the knowlege of corrupt terys, wherof ben caused fystyllys and the cures of them. Now I teche

1145 yow the verry knowlege of verry terys and yn what place they veryly spryng. Many mene wene that wepyng terys come out of the eyon, but yt is not so. For theyr yssue ys oute of the eyeledys boyth the ouer and the neþer at the ho[p. 111]les yn the lacrimal

1139. they] the H1

84

besyde the nose at the ende of the grounde of the herys, as ʒe
1150   shall euydently aspye yf ʒe wyll reuerse and turne the eyledys.
But nat forthan þere is different causes of teres whych spryng
out of the ouer eylede and whych spryng oute of the nether, ffor
tho whych come out of the nether eyelyde proceden from the
hert, eyther for sorow, drede or smart, and be caused by a
1155   maner of vyolence. But they be not durable nor abydyng, for
when the cause þerof cesyth þei sesyn. But the te[p. 112]res
whych cum oute of the hoole of the ouer lyd of the ey proceden
from the brayn and be causid of sum corrupcion of habundans,
of superfluytee of humors, and her cours ceceth not but yf the
1160   mater be pourgyd and holpen wyth oure electuaryes and cautaryes, lyke as we haue tauʒth beforne.

Now after that I haue tauʒth yow, quod he, of the hurtys that
comme to the eyon outwarde, as by strokys yn the forhede,
templys or browys, and naturally of cor[p. 113]rupte and
1165   naturale terys; now wyll I speke of the hurtys whych casually
falle vnto dyuers artifycers, as to masons, myllers, wryghtys,
smythes, and oþer. Ffor yt happyth þat sum of here fragmentys
sterte ynto there eyes vnwysyli, and rechelesly be left þeryn tyll
þei be incarnate vpon the tonycles of the ey; and the payn
1170   causeth contynually þer eyon to water so that the pacyent may
no<t> wele opon hys eye. And of thyes ʒe schal fynde som þat
haue the fragment of ston or of styke opon the lyght incarnat,
som besyde the lyght, and som betwe[p. 114]ne the blak and the
white. And of all thyes þer ys but oon maner of cure, and yt ys
1175   thus:

Make the pacyent to sytt downe and bakwarde to ley hys
hede betwene your legges. And þen doo hym shyt hys hoole eye,
and after open the sore eye and wyth a nedyll of syluer deuyde
the fragment from the place þat it ys on so sotelly and so dis-
1180   cretely that yn no wyse ʒe hurt not the tonycle, but lede it so

1171. not] no H1

softly and so sotylly yn the maner of a barbor vpon a mans berde. And so ledyng forth the nedyll by maner of shauyng, ȝe shall remoue it from the place wher it lay. [p. 115] And that doon, ȝe shall easely haue it out, and yit yn the place wher yt lay

1185 be made a grete pyt. Put into the eye of the oynement callyd the vertu youen of god whych I taugte before, and on the eye withoute lay a plaster of flaxen hurdys wyth the whyte of an egge twyes on the day and oonys of the nyght. And withyn iij dayes he shall be hoole. And yf the fragment be long þeron and

1190 be not cured on this seyd wyse, all the tonycle shall wex whyte and the pacyent shall lese hys syȝte.

Moreouer here wyll I teche yow practysers a crafte to [p. 116] take out an hawe from the eye be ensample of a cure that I dyd oonys yn Tuskayne in a cite callyd Iuk, where was brouȝt to me

1195 a man þat hade an hawe yn hys ey of the smytyng of a whete yere ouerthwart, but the nethyr ende appered outwarde on the tonycle, and yt appered as it doth when it is on a mannys fynger betwene the fleshe and the nayle. And yn thys I dyde thus indede proceden:

1200 Ffyrst y avysed me wele and wysely wher the hawe entred, and þere sotylly I kut without any trouble of the tonycle. And þan hade I rede ij nedyls [p. 117] myghtyly knytt togeder by the eyon yn maner of a twycch. Of whych oon I put the poynt vnder the hawe on the same syde wher yt went yn, and betwene the

1205 tonycle and the poynt of the toþer nedyl I put aboue the hawe. And after that sotylly I streyned them togydder, and so wyth softe wyndyng of þat oon honde and sotyll rollyng it wyth the oþer honde, I drew oute the hawe. Whych doon, anoon I put ynto the eye of the oynement aforesayd callyd virtus a deo data,

1210 twyes on the day, tyl the tonycle was sowdyd and the ey hoole. And þus do [p. 118] ȝe in lyke wyse yf ȝe wyll gett your worschyp and your pacyent helth.

It also happeneth sum tyme folkys by the styngyng of sum venemous beste yn the eye, as by waspys or attercoppys or ony

86

1215 such oþer, or with any infecte ayre that men calle blastyng,
      wherthorugh the ey wexeth so bolnyn that the pacyent may not
      opyn hys eye and the payne growyth so greueous þat he may
      haue no rest. Wherfore when ȝe see any such haue the recours
      to the gracyous herbe callyd cardus benedictus, sowthystyl. <
1220 [f. 33] *And these ben the signes to know hem, for he hathe two lyknes in*
      herselfe. Firste for it hathe litell leuys and the 2e grete leuys and brode, and
      we sayne that all ben of on complexioun and of one sauour and hauen one
      vertue, and it makethe a citren flour. > Take þerof an handful and
      stampe it and temper it [p. 119] wyth halfe the whyte of an egg,
1225 and þereof make a plaster wyth coton or flexe herdys, and the
      eye shitt ley it theron and bynd it þereto with a lynnen bend so
      that it remoue nat therfro. And so let it leye tyl it be drye, and
      after þat it is drye ley to another, and so tyl the bolnyng be
      hoole. Thys plaster ys callyd gracious for it swagyth bolnyng
1230 and yt puttyth awey blode from the eye, it swagyth the peyne
      and dystroyth the venym. And yf it happen sum tyme sodeynly
      that [that] the eye wex rede and sore brennyng, so þat [p. 120]
      the pacyent thenk þat hys eye were ful of grauel, with thys
      gracious plaster he shall ben holpen as sone as it is leyd þereon.
1235 And for thies causes and oþer, thys plaster ys callyd gracious.
          Thys þan tauȝth by thys autor, Beneuucius, the specyall hur-
      tys of eyon boyth inwardly and outwardly caused and the spe-
      cyall cures of the same. Now here yn the laste ende of thys
      booke he techeth generall medycyns, and fyrst he techyth pow-
1240 ders and after coleryous and fynally he techyth a general dyato-
      rye for al maner of such pacyentis. [p. 121]
          Ffyrst as towchyng powders, I sey to yow in the name of
      Ihesu that powder mayde of the margaryte put yn the eye
      whych hath a clowde lyke a thynne clowde sprede abrode yn the
1245 clere eyre, hit helpit it. The same doth a jasper powdryd; also yf
      the eye be red or blody, it puttyth it awey. Also cristall sotylly
      powderd doth the same that the jasper doth and also largyth the
      eye. Also a saphire powderd dooth iij thyngys in the eye: it

87

fretyth the webbe, it sharpyth the syȝte and constrenyth [p. 122]
1250 the pupyll, and clarifyeth all the eye. And after that it ys onys
entryde into the eye, it may neuer be apeyred wythout grete
hurte. Also powder of the berall fretyth away yn the eye
an<d> comfortyth all the humors. But here it ys to be markyd
þat wyth all thies powders wyth eche of them must be medled
1255 powder of suger captyu to temper and to restreyne her myȝty
vyolens, and in thys proporcyon: ij partys ben of suger and oon
of the oþer powder. And thys powder must be kept yn a boxe of
gold or of syluer, and twyes in the day [p. 123] morn and euyn
put into the eye.
1260 And not oonly of precyous stonys but also of gommys and of
oþer thyngys may be made ful holsom powders for eyon. And as
for g<u>mmys take the gomme of olyues and make þereof
powder, and þat fretyth the webbe and claryfyeth the eye.
Gomme of fenkyll doth the same and also quykenyth the visible
1265 spiritys and sharpet the lyȝth. Also gumme of bitter almondes
doth the same. And the bitter plumbes gumme the same. And
wete ȝe wel wheresoeuer the powder of the seid gummes be put
yn the eyon for the webbe or [p. 124] pannyclus, they shall
helpe and nothyng hurte.
1270 Also take suger candy and washe it wele and wype it wyth a
lynnen cloth tyl it be drye and þan powder it. Thys powder
fretyth the webbe and clarifyeth the syght and doyth many oþer
woonderful thyngys when it is entred into the eye. Also take
tutie of Alexandre sotyl and grene and powder it and medyl it
1275 wyth suger captyu, even quantitees. Thys powder restreynyth
teres and fretyth the webbe, puttyth aweye bolnyng of the eyeledys, and distroyth the ycche þereof and the blode [p. 125] of the
eyon. Also take the strenys of egg and medyll them wyth suger
captyu and bray them togheder in a brasyn morter yn the

1253. and] an H1
1262. gummys] gemmys H1

1280 maner of a sawce, and it yn a wesyll of glas and dry it all at the
son and þan powder it and þerof put yn þine eye in whych ys a
webbe, and it shall frete it wythoute peyn or violence an < d >
claryfie the syȝte. Also take the dragons roote and scrape awey
clene the berke and stampe it and wryng out the jus and medyl

1285 it wyth powder of sarcocolle yn thys maner proporcion: that is
[p. 126] ij scruples of the jows and half an vnce of the powder,
and drye yt at the son and powder it. And thys ys goode for the
webe in the eye, < [f. 35] *and in many stedis it is cleped mobilion and
in Cecile and in Calabre and in Poile, pustile. Me fyndeth many suche,*

1290 *and ye shull hele þese pacientis first whiles they ben newe and fresshe erly
and at euen, and these medicynes that ye fynde good and yproued ye shull
haue hem afore honde. Also sponge marina yclensed from sonde and ybrent
in a newe potte and make poudre, and it shall freten the clowde and
blackethe the tonicle and it clerethe the sight.* >

1295 Also an vnce of spyce callyd lignum aloes, and bren it
betwene ij bassyns so that the smoke goo not out. Whych
doone, than take 1 vnce of suger captyu and stampe it in the
ouer bassyn wyth the smoke and make a powder of them both.
After thys stampe the brend lignum aloes in the same basyn þat

1300 it was brend yn, and medyll þerewyth a drame of goode muske
and iiij dramys of amber wele smellyng. Than put [p. 127] both
powders yn on basyn and make of all oon sotyl powder. This
powder fretyth the forseyd clowde and clarifyeth the syȝte and
comforteth the vysible spirit and restrenyth teres causyd of cold

1305 humors and comforteth the brayn, lyftyng vp the eyledys, and
dystroyth the peyn of the mygreym. < [f. 35] *But wyseliche dothe
that noo asshes falle into the bacyn noþer* [f. 35v] *coles, and all shalt thou
poudry and kepe it in a boiste of siluer.* >

Also the gall of a beste callyd castor medled with the juys of

1310 an herbe clepyd morsus galline of whych herbe be ij spyces: oon
beryth a rede floure the oþer a violet floure. That whych beryth

1282. and] an H1

the rede floure ys callyd domina, the oþer [p. 128] ancilla; and
notwythstondyng this diuersytee of floures, þei ben both of oon
complexion and of oon sauor and of oon similitude, saue þat
1315   floure. Take the jous of thys herbe and put yn the thyrde proporcion and medyl it togheder and so myche of the powder of
sarcacolle that yt be as sade as past; þan dry it at the son. Than
powder it ageyn and medyll it wyth suger captyu, for it is
vyole < n > t.

1320   Also take the galle of a bere and medyll it wyth the powder of
margarytys and drye them at the soon. Than powder it [p. 129]
ageyn, and loke þer be ij partys of galle and oon of powder. Also
take the galle of an eglee and yncorporate þerwyth the powder
of iaspe and drye it yn the son. Than m < e > dyl it wyth the
1325   powder of suger captyu so that ij partys be suger and oon of
galle and of the jaspe. < [f. 36] *It shall frete the clowde and caust oute*
blode, and it shall allight and swagen the greuance of the eyȝeliddes. >

Also the oyle of olyfe put ynto the ey meruelusly fretyth the
webbe or clowde, but it ys ryȝte vyolent. Wherfore at euyn
1330   when ȝe put the oyle yn the eye, ley aboue the plaster þat is
callyd emplastrum laudabile to temper the vyolens of the oyle.
Also jowus [p. 130] of a sowre crape. Take xxti crapes ere they
be rype, confecte them wyth oure powder callyd Alexander yn
the maner of a past and drye it in the sone and powder it aȝen
1335   and medle it wyth the powder of suger captyu, dowble to the
oþer powder. Thys fretyth myghtely the sayd clowde and dys-
troyeth the rednes of the eyeledys and claryfyeth the syȝte.

Now after the doctryne of powders the autor techith dyuers
colories for diuers sekenes that fallyth yn the eyeledys and letten
1340   the syȝte and wasten the [p. 131] tonycle and lette the pacyent to
haue hys rest. And fyrst ayen rednes of the eyelyddys: take totye
of Alexander and of amatist stone, sandragon, reed corall, good

aloes, epatik euyn porcioun of eche halfe an vnce; sarcacolle, spykenard, safron of eche a drame; suger candy an vnce; cam-

1345 phir, mirrus, olibani, mastyk of eche halfe a drame; the rootys of parcely, fenel, and wormode of eche halfe an hanful. Breke all thyes thyngys togydder yn a morter and after put them yn a feyr basyn and temper þem wyth iij[p. 132] pynty[n]s of good whyte wyne and after put yt yn an erthen pott, boylle it togheder wyth

1350 a softe fyre tyll the wyne be halfe wasted. Then clense it thorugth a lynnen cloth and kepe it yn glasse and put þerof yn the pacyentys eye morn and eve tyll it be hoole.

Also aȝen the seyd sekenes of the eyledys and the rednes therof: take totye of Alexander halfe an vnce; of antemonie,

1355 erys vsti, suger captyu of eche an vnce and an halfe; and roses dryed as muche. All thyes thyngys, saue roses pouderd, put yn a erthen pote wythe [p. 133] iij pyntys of whyte wyne boyllyng wyth soft fyre tyll halfe be wastede and vse thys as the oþer beforn.

1360 Also anoþer colerie for the same: take an vnce of totye Alex- andre and xl croppys of bremel and stampe them toghedyr as it were sawce with iij pyntys of whyte wyne yn a new erthen potte. Boyle it togheder to the halfe and vse it as the toþer. Thies forseyd coleryes byth moyst preuyd for the seyd sekenes of the

1365 eyeledys, but they arn not good for the webbe yn the eye but raþer n<o>yous, for wyne ys constriktyfe [p. 134] and confyr- matyffe. And þerfore yf colerie be made wyth wyne and be put yn the eye that hath a webbe, the pacyent shall neuer be hoole nor holpyn þerewyth but rather [and] appayred.

1370 Also take totye and sarcacolle of eche halfe an vnce; roses sedys ij vnces; camphyr ij drammys. Pouder thyes togheder and boyll them in a quarte of whyte wyne to the thyrd parte, and put ij dropys yn the sore eye and it wyll put awey rednes of the eyon and restreyne teres. Also aȝen watrye eyon: yff the pacyent

1366. noyous] neyous H1: cp. it noyeþ H2/A

1375   drynk [p. 135] erely fastyng auream Alexandrinam wyth wyne, streyneth teres maruelously. Also medyll sarcacolle wyth womans mylke and dry it at the son and eftsones do the same, and than powder it and put it yn the eye whych is dusty or mysty. It cleryth well the sy3th.

1380   Now fynally drawyng to the ende of thys booke, Benuenucius spekyth to hys dysciplis concludyng thus: O 3e my dyscyples whych wyll be practysers yn cures off sore eyon, lyke as 3e haue herde me teche, [p. 136] [herde me teche] so werke. And pray god wyth laude and thankyng þat he wyll wytsayff of his spe-
1385   cyall grace to performe your cures to hys worshype and your pacyentys helth. And alwey haue awarenes in your cures to mesurable dyet of your pacyentys and to kepe them from contraryous metys tyll þei recouere perfy3te helth. That ys to wyt froo beef, gootys flech salted, from stoke fysshe, from elys, from
1390   onyons, from garlyk, from commenyng of women, from bathes, from sawcys, from grete werynes, from grete [p. 137] labour, from ouer myche wacche and fastyng. Lete hym not goo abroode yn the wynde nor yn the soon, nor loke yn no lanterne ly3te tyll they be recouered. Lete them ete rere egges wyth
1395   breed; yff þei be yong, lete them drynk water; and yff they be olde, lete them drynk wyne with water. And yff the cure tarye þat nature helpe not, yeve them fleshe of yong gootys gelded, soden and not rooste, tyll they be recouerede.

     Deo gracias.

EXPLANATORY NOTES

8–9. Deus oculorum. The usual title in the Latin manuscripts is *De probatissima arte oculorum* (VP3, f. 97; VP1, f. 245v), a title found embedded in the text itself. A full list of titles as indicated by manuscript rubrics can be found in David C. Lindberg, *A Catalogue of Medieval and Renaissance Optical Manuscripts*, Subsidia medievalia IV (Toronto: Pontifical Institute of Medieval Studies, 1975),102. One of these, *De egritudinibus oculorum*, might with sufficient abbreviation, misreading, physical damage to the manuscript, etc., have given rise to *Deus oculorum*, a title found only in H1/S. H2 is untitled, except for Hunter's title in his table of contents.

13. herde . . . foote. VP3, f. 97: Oculus est callus concauus plenus aque . . . . VP1, f. 245v, and P, f. 165v: Oculus est callus concauus rotundus plenus aque . . . . *Callus* (CL), a firm bit of flesh, came to mean frequently the pathological growth produced on the foot by rubbing, walking, etc. (MLD)

13–14. or as . . . basyn. No extant Latin manuscript gives any warrant for this phrase, nor can I see how the translator might have misconstrued the Latin texts that survive.

14. well . . . hede. VP1, f. 245v; VP3, f. 97; and P, f. 165v all read "in fronte capitis." Some other manuscripts, including evidently the one used by the translator, read "fonte capitis."

15–17. vysyble . . . withoute. The theory of vision on which this description rests is described in the Introduction, p. 9.

27. Johannitius. The ninth-century Arabic physician Hunain ibn Ishaaq was known to western Europe as Johannitius. The anatomical information repeated here can be found in his *Ysagoge* or commentary on Galen. See Introduction, pp. 11–12, for further discussion.

32–35. The . . . yolow. A curious description of eye colour, but all Latin manuscripts agree on the first three, *niger*, *subalbidus*, and *varius*.

The fourth colour is usually *glaucus*, grey, evidently miscopied by the translator or already present as *blancus* in his Latin manuscript. I am not sure how to translate these colours into modern English, but perhaps dark brown, pale blue, hazel, and grey would be suitable approximations.

35-37. The . . . egge. Modern terminology retains both the vitreous and the albugineous humours, though aqueous humour is often found instead of albugineous. English terminology now prefers "lens" for *cristallinus*, though French *cristallin*, and Italian *cristallino* retain the older term.

40. anothomie. Frequently in medieval medical treatises, anatomy means no more than systematic knowledge of the human body and carries no implication of dissection. None of the extant Latin manuscripts carries the explicit statement that anatomy means cutting a cadaver.

43-46. Yif . . . consumed. The argument, from H2, is truncated. Benvenutus claims that if there were seven tunics, then a perforated eye would not leak out the humours from within. But since a perforated eye usually does leak out its humours, he concludes that there must be fewer tunics protecting it. Here is a text from one of the manuscripts with the Extended Anatomy (punctuation added): Si tunice oculorum sunt septem secundum Johannitium, ergo cum prima tunica frangitur tota substantia oculi non deuastatur. Sed quia secundum nos non sunt nisi due, et cum prima frangitur tota substantia oculi deuastatur et oculus consumitur cum suis humoribus. Alia uero est perforata propter quod humores oculorum non possunt retineri postquam prima tunica est fracta. VV, f. 288v.

46-47. The . . . variaunce. Despite calling this the tonicle, he is here describing the iris, which he may think of as the uvea tunic.

54-92. The theory that seeks to align eye colour with acuity and durability of sight and with the depth of the cristalline humour within the eye seems original with Benvenutus.

60. humors. That is, the cristalline humour, the lens.

65. meuable. Apparently a misreading of *mediocriter*, as in *mediocriter niger* (VP1, f. 245v), light black or grey.

94

66–67. obtalmie . . . panniclus. For these illnesses see lines 360–569.

71. hangyn. This translates *pendent* (sunt varii et pendent in albedinem [VP1, f. 246]), as in many Latin manuscripts. But cp. VP3, f. 97v: et tendunt ad albedinem.

73–74. bendyng humors of teris. P, f. 165v: magis superveniunt lacrime et reuma. VP1, f. 246: magis latericie [sic] et reuma perueniunt. VP3, f. 97v: multis [?] superveniunt scilicet reuma et lacrime. It is difficult to see how the translator arrived at "bendyng."

95. naye. Formed by metanalysis in a similar manner to adder or newt: the *n* of the indefinite article in the phrase "an ey" became separated from the article and attached itself to the following vowel. The form then persisted independent of the indefinite article, though apparently without becoming standard.

97–106. Wherfore . . . vitreus. These lines describe the three humours of the eye, especially how they feel to the touch. The "maner of holwenes in the ouer partie of optici nerffe" (VP3, f. 97v: Est quedam concauitas in summitate nerui optici) is the eyeball itself.

99. yelwisshe. VP1, f. 246: glaucose. P, f. 166: glaucosa. Properly greyish, but see MLD 2 *glaucus* (sense 3), where yellowish is an attested meaning, though not with reference to the eye.

100. not. The three distinctions in the humours (nature, name, and feeling) require a "not" before figure, but not all Latin manuscripts have it there. P, f. 166, and VP3, f. 97v, have a *non*; VP1, f. 246, lacks it.

108–13. Therfor . . . humour. The humoural theory of physiology assigns two characteristics to each humour, by making permutations of cold/hot and moist/dry. The three humours of the eye lend themselves less symmetrically to the four qualities. The description works from the deepest humour, the albugineous, outwards to a point where the moistness of the sanguine humour in the eyelids can offset the dryness of the neighboring vitreous humour. Modern ophthalmology makes the vitreous humour the deepest.

113–15. sithen . . . brayne. Gummosity translates the Latin *gummositas*, gumminess (MLD), but I do not know what to make of the physiology.

120-23. a cateracte . . . humor. Ancient and medieval ophthalmology thought of a cataract as a sort of corrupt humour or water that descended within the eye between the cristalline humour and the tunics. Modern ophthalmology holds that it is a clouding of the lens itself.

131. celestyal. That is, blue.

144. with his signe. Awkward translation of *signa*, "symptoms." VP1, f. 246v: et postquam sunt completi, hec sunt signa: paciens nihil videt nisi . . . .

155-57. Sarazyns . . . ey3e. Benvenutus appears to have had no Arabic, and "amesarca" is probably a distortion produced by manuscript transmission. See Introduction, p. 13, for further discussion.

184. it. That is, the cataract.

191. thyrllyng. Translator's error for wrything, that is twisting to and fro. VP1, f. 247: et postea plane extrahas acum sicud misisti torquendo cum digitis tuis.

197. remeue. That is, replace, renew.

258-60. And . . . rewe. Cp. the Latin: in hieme vero semper bibat vinum calidum in quo ponatur salvia et ruta (VP1, f. 247). The translator may have mistaken *vero* for *non*.

284-85. þat . . . sy3te. Gloss on pyupyl (= pupil), evidently added by the translator.

287-88. And . . . wombe. Translates, but not terribly well: dicimus quod accidit eis in utero materno per aliqua corruptione que duratur ibi (VP1, f. 247v).

304. that . . . mortifyed. Added presumably by the translator to gloss *opylate*. VP1, f. 248, reads: nerui optici sunt ita opilati et mortificati.

313-14. lyke . . . renewed. Both the Latin and the English are obscure here. VP1, f. 248, reads: quasi in colore veridi sicud lipitudo que est in aquis multis. VP3, f. 99v: in colore veridi sicut lippitudo que est in aquis in multis locis.

315-16. litell and lytell. VP3, f. 99v: ista species cataractarum incurabilium non paulatim venit sed subito descendit et ita repente quod . . . . The translator evidently missed the *non*, making the two clauses of his sentence contradictory.

336. yt . . . vp. VP3, f. 99v: facit palpebras reuersare. That is, it may cause an everted eyelid, a lower lid that droops and does not close properly.

366–67. occasyon . . . panycles. That is, ophthalmia may lead to pannicles, though the Latin does not say this. VP1, f. 248: vnde propter hoc obtalmia duratur temporibus illis et hac occasione obtalmie generantur in oculis.

371. blaknes. Here, the iris. VP1, f. 248v: circumcirca tunicas nigredinem oculorum.

393–95. Knowe . . . peyne. VP1, f. 248v: sciatis karissimi quod propter custodias et curam malam quam stulti faciunt ignorantes artes oculorum sequentes errores cum medicinis suis committunt et adiungunt dolorem ad dolorem. VP3, f. 100: vnde sciatis karissimi propter malam custodiam et malam curam quam stulti multi medicini faciunt ignorantes artem et sequentes errorem cum medicinis suis adiungunt dolorem super dolorem.

402. syȝte. That is, site, location. VP1, f. 248v: oculi cum tota concauitate extra palpebras apparit.

413. dyolibanum. Recipe lines 244–48.

415. puluis nabetys. More properly, pulvis nabatis. Literally, Arabic powder. Recipe lines 515–23.

417–18. puluis Alexandrini. Identified in the Latin manuscripts as the remedy for the third phlegmatic illness. VP1, f. 250, reads: hoc facto impleas totum oculum plenum de puluere alexander sine ulla mixtione. Cp. line 633 below. It seems to be sugar worked with a pestle until it becomes a fine powder.

474. But yf. = unless.

488–89. rownde . . . cautaryes. He recommends a tubular cautery rod, such that the round end actually does the cauterizing. Benvenutus alludes often to his treatise or lecture on cauteries, but it has never been identified.

496. puluis nabetis. More properly, pulvis nabatis. Recipe at lines 515–23.

520. nabiatis. More properly nabatis. That is, sugar. There is consid-

erable confusion over the names and properties of the various powders mentioned, not only here but also in the Latin manuscripts. The following note is appended to the treatise in VV, f. 179: Nota quod puluis alexandrinus potest esse compositus nabatis cum fumo ligni aloe — puluis nabatis est simplex. Uel puluis alexandrinus potest esse puluis benedictus qui ex sarcocolla, sed dubium est quia non fit alia notitia [?] in libro. Sed uterque puluis bonus est sed vltimus est magis ponderans, et credo quod vltimus sit melior quia magis corrodit carnositatem. Sed caute: consideretur quantitas carnositatis vt si fuerit multa pondus [?] sarcocolla. Si modico nabatis, uel compositus uel simplex, et hec dubitatio surgit ex capitulo loquente de humiditatibus superuenientibus ex causa flegmatica capitulo tertio [punctuation added]. The third phlegmatic illness is described at lines 621–50.

525–26. plastre . . . applis. Recipe at lines 498–500.

533. zucre . . . Alexandri. This is probably loaf sugar, and the uncertainty of its name probably reflects its relatively recent introduction from Arabic countries to Europe. Often the name nabatis (or nabetis) stands on its own, as does candi, and the name Alexander applied adjectively seems to mean "made of sugar."

556–57. neysshe of the heued. Literally, the soft part of the head; the back of the neck? VP1, f. 250: in mollicu capitis. VP3, f. 102: in mollicie capitis.

563. it. That is, the cure.

568. they. That is, the other medicines that are violent.

579. they. That is, the patients.

580. þei. That is, the hairs.

585–86. Wherfore . . . thus. That is, otherwise than the method just described of pulling the hairs out. Benvenutus's recommended procedure follows.

587–94. Take . . . þem. This description is not terribly clear, either in Latin or in English. Barrough's attempt to clarify leads the S scribe to a contemptuous marginal note: "Note here howe without sence Barrowe hath penned it in his booke willing to bind the needles at both þe endes, before you take vpp þe skynn" (f. 40). Perhaps it is intended that the physician, after threading both needles, should leave the thread slack while he binds the pointed ends tightly together. Then using the needles like a longitudinal clamp, he catches between them a bit of flesh from the underside of the upper eyelid and, using the previously threaded thread, binds the other end of the needles together, tightly enough so that they will within a short time cut through the flesh that has been caught up. But I cannot conceive how in the midst of this procedure the patient should manage to open and close her eyes.

598. puluis nabetis. Recipe lines 515–23.

612. soft . . . hede. Cp. note at 556–57. Perhaps the back of the neck?

614. pouder of candye. No recipe given. Perhaps just sugar reduced to fine powder with nothing added.

616. pulule Iherosolomitane. Recipe lines 165–69.

618. diaolibanum Salernitanum. Recipe lines 244–48.

633. powder of candie. Cp. note at line 614. There is no recipe for powder of candy given in the text.

636. and xv days after. That is, every day for fifteen days.

644. puluis benedictus. Recipe lines 378–80

674. plaster gracious. Recipe lines 637–39.

677. colerium Alexandrinum. No recipe for this collyrium is given in the treatise. VP3, f. 103, also recommends it without giving a recipe.

710. the gowte and the palsye. The sense of the Latin is a touch of the palsy. VP1, f. 251: guttam paralisis. VP3, f. 103v: guttam in palpebris. Gutta can mean an inflamation; see MLD s.v. *gutta* (sense 6).

760. forsaide gumme. The Latin recipe calls for fennel gum, *gummi feniculi* (VP1, f. 251v), instead of fennel seed. The lengthy praise of fennel gum that follows (764–71) suggests that the H2 scribe may have misread the Latin when he wrote *sede* in line 758.

781–82. the same. That is, he sees four of them.

785–86. lectuarye . . . aperytyff. Cp. the recipe with the same name at lines 730–40. And note also that Benvenutus assigns another name to it at line 802.

816. succum liqueritiae. Cp. Latin: succi liqueris (VP3, f. 104v).

854. puluis nabetis. Properly pulvis nabatis. Recipe lines 515–23.

882. citramowtayns. Literally those living this side of the mountains, presumably on the Italian side of the Alps. VP1, f. 252, and VP3, f. 105, identify these same people as the *vltramarini*. Other Latin manuscripts call them the *ultramontani*.

888. ʒelkys. Probably should read "whites," as Benvenutus always recommends egg white as a dressing for both diseases and injuries to the eye. VP1, f. 252v, and VP3, f. 105, read: vitella ouorum.

894. And . . . plaster. VP3, f. 105, reads: dicimus quod tria facit. VP1, f. 252v, reads: et dicimus quod tria facit. The translator goes on to say the three things the ointment does, and no doubt he misread the Latin in introducing the three.

900. is . . . roost. Cp. Latin: cocta bene donec sint mollia (VP1, f. 252v). Evidently the translator mistook *mollia* for *meliora*, and then did his best with the phrase.

914-15. vnguentum alabastrum. Recipe lines 445-56.

922. eylydys reuersed. Probably an everted eyelid, a lower lid that hangs too far open, so that its inner surface is visible.

948. smale . . . before. That is, the "lytyl pylowe" of lines 926-27. Cp. VP1, f. 252v: postquam fecimus cum albumini oui et super cicatrice ponebamus pulluillos illos (as in lines 926-27), and f. 253: quo facto habeatis polluillos sicud in alijs curis de reuersatis palpebris.

956. muri or wulgalpus. Cp. VP1, f. 253: a multis vocatur muru et volgariter cersu et multi vocant ipsum volgariter fungum. VP3, f. 105v: in multis locis vocatur muri et vvlgariter cersu uel secundum alios et vvlgariter dicitur fungus. "Wulgalpus," which occurs in no Latin manuscript, may be a misreading of *vulgariter*.

962. vnguentum subtile. Recipe lines 909-11.

986. founde be practyffe. Cp. VP1, f. 253: de virtute a deo data a nobis inventa.

986. virtus a deo data. Recipe lines 1001-3.

987-88. But . . . past. This appears to be a sentence inserted at random (?) with little apparent basis in the Latin. Cp. VP1, f. 253: Sed si tunica sit fracta ponatis intus in oculo de virtute a deo data a nobis inventa (et ita vocamus eam quia factus est de generibus ouorum sicud inferius dicemus) bis in die et semel in nocte. Et propter hoc non dimittatur quendam bombacem intinctum in clara oui; super oculum clausum usque ad predictum terminum ponatis, et interim sepius vngatur supercilia fronte et tympora pacientis de vnguento nostro alabastro (punctuation added).

1018. as . . . cataract. That is, at lines 165–210.

1028. this plaster. That is, the plaster made of cumin and wax used by the lewde leches of line 1020.

1044–45. but . . . suppose. Cp. lines 1077–83, the brief missing portion on festeles.

1050. lasse . . . place. The outer corner of the eye, a translation of lacrimale minoris.

1060–63. Wherfor . . . seiþ. That is, if the pupil contracts and dilates with the increase and lessening of light, then some sight remains in the eye.

1060–61. balle of the eyȝe. Translates *pupilla* (VP1, f. 254).

1071–74. in . . . doynges. These other causes are contrasted with blows around the eyes. They are less apt to cause this type of blindness than the blows, though the Latin is a bit more ambiguous: omnis nerui optici opilantur: primo per oculationem [?] sue [sic] opilatione possimus intelligere multa ieiunia et vigilias; secunda accio [= actio] fit per multas angustias et planctum lacrimarum et multas verberaciones capitis et fatigationes corporis et similiter; accidit multis per nimium coitum quibusdam, et per multum legere et scribere et ad huc nerui optici opilantur similiter; et magis opilantur illi qui sunt percussi sicud diximus supra . . . et magis opilantur in istis quam in aliquibus istorum (VP1, f. 254).

1104–1107. of the . . . destroyed. The translation is a bit awkward. Cp. the Latin: quia nerui oculorum habent viam iuxta nasum proprie ubi illi stolidi medici faciunt cauterium et <faciendo?> [seciendo, manuscript] illum ignem nerui desiccantur (VP1, f. 254).

1110. peletys of Ierusalem. Recipe lines 165–69.

1121. coresey . . . powder. Lines 1242–1337 supply recipes for several powders, all of which have certain corrosive properties, but none of which seems exactly what is wanted here — that is, a powder designed specifically against fistulas.

1142. electuarium mirabile. Recipe lines 690–702.

1186. vertu . . . god. Recipe lines 1001–3.

1194. Iuk. That is, Lucca in Tuscany. Cp. Latin: in quadam civitate que vocatur luca (VP1, f. 255).

1196–97. but . . . tonycle. Cp. Latin: ita quod capita ariste non apparebat super tunicam (VP1, f. 255). Evidently the translator overlooked the *non*.

1209. virtus . . . data. Recipe lines 1001–3.

1219–25. gracyous . . . herdys. Recipe for this gracious plaster is also given at lines 637–39.

1250–52. And . . . hurte. Nothing appears in the Latin that might serve as a basis for this sentence.

1252. Also . . . eye. The Latin has a direct object here, *nebulam*, a web (VP1, f. 255v). Perhaps the translator confused "away" with "a web" and omitted the latter.

1255. suger captyu. Translates *zuccerum captivum*, a term Benvenutus never explains. Most other manuscripts have *zuccero captivo*: VP3, f. 108v: zuccero caffethino; VP1, f. 255v: zuccero cathino; VP2, f. 310v: zuccero capituo; VR, f. 58v: zuccere cattiuo.

1270. suger candy. Cp. Latin: Recipe ergo zuccerum nabatis arabicum secundum nos vocatum candi (VP3, f. 109). Recipe zuccarum nabetis secundum arabes sed secundum [no gap in manuscript] vocatur candi (VP1, f 255v).

1288. it. That is, the web in the eye.

1295–98. Also . . . both. Cp. the recipe for puluis nabatis, lines 515–23. The musk and amber are additional here.

1331. emplastrum laudabile. Recipe lines 822–26.

1354. antemonie. Probably not pure antimony, but see Jacalyn Duffin and Pierre René, "Anti-moine; 'Anti-biotique': the Public Fortunes of the Secret Properties of Antimony Potassium Tartrate (Tartar Emetic)," *Journal of the History of Medicine and Allied Sciences* 46 (1991), 440–456.

GLOSSARY

Included here are words apt to be unfamiliar to readers of, say, Chaucer or Langland. Words spelled in variable Middle English orthography are usually not listed. Though no attempt has been made to provide a full concordance, at least a one-line reference is provided for all but the most common words. In alphabetizing *v* and *u* are treated as the same letter, as are *i, j*, and vocalic *y*. Yogh is placed after *g*, thorn after *t*. Headwords in Latin are italicized.

accacioun (152) a nonce word of no meaning; see Introduction, p. 41.

accesse (749) n., an attack of illness, fever, ague (MED); cp. axesse

acurye (277) adj., fr L *acuaria*, fr L *acus*, needle; of or pertaining to a needle

agaryk (354) agaricus (815) n., probably a type of fungus used medicinally (MED); polyporus officinalis (Hunt)

aye (102) n., var. of ei, egg; pl. eyron (MED)

akthe (547) n., ache (MED)

albigenius (36), albugineus (95) and other spellings, adj., fr L, pertaining to the albigeneous humour in the eye

alexander (791) n., the herb horse parsley (MED, Hunt); poss. cucurbita alexandrina, colocynth (Hunt); see also the note to line 533

algattis (262) adv., in any event, nevertheless (MED)

almandys (793) n., almonds (MED)

aloes (167) n., aloe, either the tree or the juice or resin of the tree (MED)

amatist (1342) n., the semi-precious stone amethyst (MED)

amber (1301) n., fossilized pine resin, amber (MED)

amesarca (156) n., fr Arabic, cataract; cp. VP1, f. 246v: amesaros; VP3, f. 98: ylmesarac

ana (353) adv., fr ML, fr Gr, in an equal amount (MED)

103

and (passim) conj., and (MED sense 1); conj., if (MED sense 5)

anglice (49) adv., in English

annes (694) n., the herb anise, also dill (MED); perhaps dog's or hog's
    fennel (Hunt)

anothomie (40) n., anatomy; usually implying systematic knowledge of
    the body and its parts, not necessarily dissection

antemonie (1354) n., antimony; probably not pure antimony

aperytyf (726) adj., (medicinal) designed to open up (MLD s.v.
    aperitivus)

appayred (1369) adj., injured, damaged, worse (MED)

appell (49) appill (154) n., pupil (of the eye) (MED appel sense 6)

aqua (156) n., water

Arabies (156) n., Arabs

aranea (31) adj., the name Johannitius gives to one of the tunics or
    coverings of the eye

ars (162) n., art

aspye (1150) v., notice, observe (MED aspien sense 6b)

attercoppys (1214) n., spiders (MED)

aureum alexandrinum (1375) n., perhaps an error for aurum alexan-
    drinum? which in turn is perhaps a potion with finely powdered gold
    in suspension? cp. aurum potabile

axesse (468) n., an attack of illness, ague (MED); cp. accesse

balsami (815) n., balm (MED s.v. balsamum); gum of the balsam tree
    (Hunt)

Barbarye (681) territory of the Berbers in North Africa

basylycon (694) n., the herb basil (MED); snake root (Hunt)

bawson (756) n., badger (MED s.v. bausene), translates the Latin *taxo*
    or *tasso*, some mss *castor* (VP1, f. 251v: casso. VP3, f. 104: taxo)

berall (1252) n., the semi-precious stone beryl (MED s.v. berels)

betymes (346) betyme (665) adv., early, promptly (MED s.v. bitime)

blancus (34) adj., white; probably an error for *glaucus* (see note to line 34)

blastyng (1215) adj., blowing heavily (MED); carrying infection?

bleryed (337) adj., bleary eyed; perhaps a specific pathological condition (MED s.v. blerinesse)

blysse (175) v., bless, cross (sc. oneself) (MED s.v. blessen sense 5)

boiste (1308) n., a jar or box (MED)

boystious (577) adj., crude, unskilled, ignorant (MED)

bolne (373) bolleyn (652) adj., swollen (MED s.v. bellen)

bray (825) v., to break a substance into small fragments by chopping, crushing, grinding, etc. (MED s.v. braien)

brasyn (760) brasym (379) adj., made of copper, bronze, or brass (MED)

bremell (445) bremyl (868) n., bramble or brier, blackberry bush (MED)

brynnyng (333) adj., burning (MED s.v. brennen)

brusces (731) n., brushwood, shrub (MED); butcher's broom, knee holly (Hunt)

bruse (824) v., to squash or mash (MED s.v. brisen sense 3(b))

bruser (228) adj., wounded, bruised (by analogy from MED brisure, n.)

Calabre (1289) n., Calabria, region of southern Italy

camamyl (263) n., the herb camomile (MED)

campher (696) n., camphor (MED)

candy (604) n., crystallized cane sugar (MED)

capyllys veneris (732) n., maidenhair fern (MED)

cardomomi (692) n., the spice cardamom (MED); watercress, garden cress (Hunt)

cardus benedictus (638) n., the herb sowthistle, blessed thistle, groundsel, our lady's thistle (Hunt s.v. sowthistle)

carnosyte (622) n., a mass or knot of flesh (MED)

carnous (622) adj., of a pathological growth resembling flesh (MED)

caruy (791) n., the herb carvi, caraway (Hunt)

castor (246) castorij (691) n., dried pineal gland of the European beaver (MED); translates castorei (VP3, f. 99), genitive of castoreum, a medicine made from the scent gland of the beaver (MLD)

catapucie minoris (354) n., the herb caper spurge (MED)? MED and Hunt agree that catapucie is caper spurge, but neither deals with *catapucie minoris*

cauterye (487) See Introduction, p. 17

Cecile (1289) n., Sicily, the island off the southern coast of Italy

celle (16) n., a ventricle of the brain; see Introduction, p. 8

cerase (793) n., cerasa, cherry (Hunt)

charge (174) v., instruct, direct (MED s.v. chargen sense 5)

chasteyn (249) chesteyne (704) n., chestnut (MED)

cicatryce (1136) n., scar (MED)

Cicile (881) n., Sicily, the island off the southern coast of Italy

cycorye (732) n., the herb chicory or poss. heliotrope (MED); chicory or marigold (Hunt)

cynomom (792) n., the spice cinnamon (Hunt s.v. cinnamomum)

citramowntayns (882) n., a nonce word (?), translating L *citramontani*, presumably those living to the north but still on the Italian side of the Alps

citren (1223) adj., reddish or brownish yellow (MED)

cytryne (408) n., the herb celandine? poss. the African citrus tree? (MED); houseleek (Hunt s.v. sticados)

clouys (244) n., the spice cloves (MED)

colerium (338) n., collyrium, a type of medicine designed to go into the eye

colerium ruborum (867) n., a type of collyrium

colery (338) n., collyrium, a medicine designed to be put directly into the eye; plurals: coleryous (1240) coloryus (624)

color (330) n., yellow bile, one of the four humours (MED s.v. colre)

comyn (1021) commyn (1025) n., the spice cumin (MED)

commenyng (260) n., sexual intercourse (MED s.v. communen sense 4)

complexioun (107) n., nature (of a person or thing) resulting from a particular blending of the four humours (MED)

confect (169) v., to prepare by combining ingredients (MED)

confermed (144) adj., firmly established, fully developed (MED s.v. confermen sense 8)

confortatiuus (280) adj., invigorating, strengthening, soothing (MED) congelid (153) congyeld (121) adj., coagulated, thickened (MED)

coniunctiua (32) adj., one of the tunics coverning the eye; see Introduction, pp. 11–12

consolydatyfe (1006) adj., of a medicine, having the property to promote healing, close a wound, etc. (MED)

consowdyn (911) v., to heal, to promote healing (MED)

constriktyfe (1366) adj., of a medicine, having the property to thicken or restrain a discharge or distention (MED)

contrarius (252) adj., harmful (MED); harmful to a particular condition

coolore (714) n., the choleric humour, yellow bile (MED)

corall (1342) n., Mediterranean coral (MED)

coresey (1121) adj., corrosive, having the property of destroying organic tissue (MED)

corne (429) n., a grain or seed of a cereal (MED)

cornea (32) adj., one of the tunics covering the eye; see Introduction, pp. 11–12

cornellys (430) n., plural of kernel

cowrs (1131) n., here, the flow of pus from an infection (MED s.v. cours sense 6)

crabbys (498) n., crab apples (MED)

crape (1332) n., grape, translates *uva* (VP1, f. 256)

creature (432) n., Neapolitan name for the first type of pannicle

cristallinus (36) cristallyne (54) adj., L and Eng, one of the three humours in the eye; see Introduction, p. 13

croppys (445) n., the parts of a medicinal herb except the roots; i.e., leaves, blossoms, berries, etc. (MED)

crude (121) crudded (154) n. and adj., coagulated or thickened substance (MED)

cubibys (409) n., the herb cubeba (Hunt)

cure (483) n., medical care, treatment (MED)

decoccioun (263) n., a mixture of herbs or other made by applying heat, cooking (MED)

deuyed (924) v., divided (scribal omission?)

dylle (168) n., the herb dill (OED)

diolibanum (241) n., a compound herbal medicine

discoloratam (51) adj., lit. without colour; the name Benvenutus gives to the second of the two tunics he acknowledges

discolurde (52) adj., lit. without colour; a translation of *discolorata*

disgregat (77) adj., shedding tears (MED)

disparbolyd (84) adj., of the eyes, watering, shedding tears (MED)

dyssauerd (401) adj., disunited, separated (MED)

dyssolued (77) adj., weakened (MED)

dissouatyfe (1034) adj., weakening, destroying (MED)

dystemperd (122) adj., disposed or arranged (MED)

distemperance (971) n., imbalance of the four humours (MED)

distourblethe (1056) v., injures, harms (MED)

domyne (365) n., power (translated in text)

dominium (223) n., lordship; see Introduction, p. 41

down (passim) adv. and prep., down; sometimes past part., done

draganti (793) n., dragonwort (MED); adderwort, bistort [*dragantea*], charlock, wild mustard, wild radish [*dragancia*] (Hunt)

dragons roote (1283) n., a herb, possibly dragon arum (Hunt)

dram (168) n., a unit of weight, ca. 1/8 of an ounce (MED)

eelys (253) elys (646) n., eels (MED)

eglee (1323) n., eagle (MED)

eyre (364) n., air (MED)

eyren (558) n., eggs; pl. of ei, fr OE aeg, largely replaced by ON egg (MED)

electuarie (241) n., a liquid medicine to be swallowed, usually containing honey (MED)

emplastrum laudabile (821) n., a type of plaster or thick salve

encorporate (448) adj., thoroughly mixed into a uniform mass (MED)

epatica (167) epatyk (662) n., the herb liverwort (MED)

erys vsti (1355) n., an herb? erustrix, bramble? (Hunt); cp. VP1, f. 256v: ex istis 1 oz; VP3, f. 110: eris usti; VP2, f. 313v: eris usti; VR, f. 34 aeris usti erthyn (342) adj., made of baked or fired clay (MED)

esule (408) n., a plant of the spurge genus (MED) *esule minoris* (730), not listed in MED or Hunt

eufrasie (789) n., the herb eufrasy (MED), eyebright (Hunt)

fantastical (16) adj., pertaining to the anterior ventricle of the brain; see Introduction, p. 8

fat (262) n., here = vat, tub

fecche (1117) n., i.e., vetch (MED); here translates *cicer*, chick pea; see Hunt s.v. cicerum

fenel (694) fenkyl (447) n., the herb or vegetable fennel (MED)

fer (319) prep., for (MED)

ferforth (452) adv., to such an extent (MED)

fistule (1080) festeles (1046) n., fr *fistula*; an infection, a septic wound, a boil (MED)

flaxe (193) n., flax, i.e., the linen cloth made from flax (MED s.v. flex sense 3)

flaxen (381) adj., made of linen (MED)

fleyng (779) adj., flying (MED)

flyes (779) n., any flying insects (MED)

flume (268) flewme (330) n., phlegm, the phlegmatic humour, one of the body's four fluids or humours (MED)

fluxe (574) n., the flow of a fluid from the body, e.g., tears (MED)

forme (172) n., a bench (MED forme sense 3(c))

forþan (292) adv. and conj., on that account, because, since, so that (MED)

forwhy (149) adv. and conj., because (MED for-whi sense 5)

frakyn (434) n., freckle (MED s.v. fraknes)

freten (1293) v., to corrode, destroy, esp. bodily tissue (MED)

fro (87, 180, 183) adv. either from or fro, as in to and fro; or sometimes conj., for (MED)

fume (265) n., vapour, smoke (MED)

fumous (92) adj., vapour-like, smoky (MED)

109

fumosytee (133) n., vapour, exhalation generated by the body's humours (MED)

furosite (548) n., furiousness, suddenness (MED)

furowre (719) n., wrath, fury (MED)

gendred (92) adj., caused, brought about (MED)

ghetys (253) n., goat's (i.e., goat's flesh or meat) (MED s.v. got)

glayre (825) n., egg white (MED)

gommys (1260) n., gums, i.e., resins exuded by a tree or shrub (MED)

gowte (710) n., an inflamation of some sort in the eye (MLD s.v. gutta sense 6)

grana cytemorum (794) n., quince seed

grauelous (954) adj., of flesh, lumpy like gravel (MED)

grene (461) greynes (430) n., grain, kernel (MED)

greynous (655) adj., grainy, like grains (cp. MED s.v. grain sense 4)

groos (133) adj., thick, heavy (MED)

grounde (1149) n., base from which the eyelashes grow (MED s.v. ground sense 4(c))

gummarum Arabici (793) n., Arabic gum, resin from a species of acacia (MED)

gumme (passim) n., resin from various trees and shrubs (MED)

gummosite (114) n., a nonce word translating L *gummositas*, gumminess (MLD), of uncertain anatomical significance

guttam serenam (283) n., technical term for amaurosis (OED); see Introduction, p. 14

guttatici (431) n., regional term for the first type of pannicle

hangyn (71) translates *pendent*; see note to line 71

hawe (1193) n., the awn or beard of an ear of grain (OED); MED s.v. haue n. (3) wrongly defines this as ungula or tumour

henbane (696) n., the herb henbane (MED s.v. hen 2)

hennys grece (909) n., chicken fat (MED)

herdis (193) n., flax, the coarse part of flax (MED s.v. herd n. (3)); linen?

heuyd (548) n., the head (MED s.v. hed)

high (766) adj., strong, efficacious (MED s.v. heigh sense 3(a))

hylwort (789) n., the herb pennyroyal (MED)

humeris benedictum (880) n., one of the regional names for a sty

humor (858) n., any liquid; specifically one of the four humours (sanguine, phlegmatic, choleric, melancholic) of the body or one of the
three humours (albugineous, crystalline, vitreous) of the eye; any
pathological fluid in the body (e.g., pus) or the resulting swelling

jasper (1245) iaspe (1324) n., the precious stone jasper (MED)

id est (109) that is

iherafrumaxyn (658) n., Arabic name, as reported here, for the fourth
phlegmatic illness, scabies in the eye; cp. VP1, f. 250v: larafrumaxin;
VP3, f. 103: minaxium

Iherusolimitane (166) adj., of Jerusalem

ymeynte (1081) adj., mixed (MED s.v. imengen)

impertynent (394) adj., inappropriate, unsuitable (MED)

incarnate (476) adj., (medical) usually applied to a pathological growth
that has become firmly joined to the normal flesh, e.g., a tumour in
the eye

insysyon (1112) incytion (40) n., incision, a cut made in surgery (MED)

yndegest (141) adj., of food or drink, undigested (MED)

yroted (157) adj., rotten, corrupt (MED)

Ysagogys (28) n., a book title; see note to line 27

ysop (695) n., the herb hyssop (MED s.v. isope)

jus (355) jows (169) n., juice, sap (MED s.v. jus)

kynde (100) n., nature (MED)

lacrymal (671) n., the corner of the eye (MED)

lacrimabili minore (837) n., the outer corner of the eye, toward the ear
(error for lacrimale)

laten (213) n., latoun, an alloy of copper, tin, and other metals (MED) laurei (692) n., (error for?) laurel, translates *folium lauri* (VP1, f. 251), laurel leaf, bay leaf

leche (27) n., physician or surgeon (MED)

lectuarye (467) n., medicine to be swallowed; cp. electuary (MED)

ledder (590) n., leather, skin of a living person (MED s.v. lether sense 2)

lesse (303) conj., unless

let (840) v., hinder, impede (MED s.v. letten)

letuce (817) n., the vegetable lettuce (Hunt)

lewde (147) adj., ignorant, unskilled (MED s.v. leud)

lycoryse (789), n., liquorice, the dried root of the plant glycyrrhiza glabra (MED)

lyght (50) n., light, as of the sun or a lantern; the faculty of sight (MED)

lygnum aloes (815) n., the tree aquilaria agalocha or its wood (MED)

ly3tely (217) adv., easily (MED)

lynet (1137) n., lint made by scraping linen (MED)

lyst (892) n., strip, bit (of cloth) (MED s.v. liste n. (2))

long (953) n., lung (MED)

macys (167) n., the outer covering of nutmeg (MED)

maladictam (883) n., regional name for a sty

Marchia (620) n., the Marches, a region of central Italy

margaryte (1243) n., pearl (MED)

marina (1292), adj., of the sea, marine

mastic (167) masticys (409) n., sing. and pl., the resin exuded from the mastik tree (MED)

matrice (466) n., the uterus, womb (MED)

me (299) indef. pron., one, they, etc. (MED)

medlyd (200) adj., mixed, blended (MED)

Messana (1011) n., Messina, city of Sicily

metis (133) n., food, nourishment of any sort (MED)

meueable (65) adv., a lighter shade (of black), grey; translates VP1, f. 245v: mediocriter niger; VP3, f. 97, niger mediocriter

mygrym (137) mygreyme (708) n., migraine headache (MED)

myleseed (429) n., millet seed (MED)

milie (459) n., millet (MED)

milys (429) n., L? millet

myrabolanys (408) n. pl., fruits of any of several species of Terminalia (MED)

mirabolys cytryne (813) n., fruit of the Terminalia citrina (MED)

mirre (815) mirrus (1345) n., myrrh, resin from the tree Commiphora abyssinica (MED)

mytigatyf (726) adj., soothing, palliative (MED)

mo (650) adj., more (MED)

mobilion (1288) n., regional name for a web in the eye

molifi (890) v., soften, make into a paste (MED)

morsus galline (1310) n., the herb chickweed starwort, also common pimpernell (MED)

morter (760) n., a mortar, a bowl used for grinding and mixing ingredients (MED)

mortifyed (304) adj., deadened, benumbed (MED)

mortyficat (1121) adj., perhaps synonymous with coresey (q.v.)

mowen (158) v., may, are capable of (MED)

mugworte (355) n., the herb mugwort (artemesia vulgaris) or wormwood (artemesia absinthium) (MED)

muri (956) n., regional name for an infection in the inner corner of the eye

muske (696) n., probably some aromatic sap obtained from a tree or shrub (MED)

nabiatis (520) adj., (usually nabatis) Arabic, of Arabic origin; here = sugar

naye (95) n., egg; see note to line 95

nemenyd (766) v., to specify, to speak of by name (MED)

neppe (695) n., turnip (MED)

nerffe (50) neruus (16) neruis (114) n., sing. and pl., nerve, nerves (MED)

neysshe (556) n., something soft, the softest part of a thing (MED)

nesshe (535) adj., soft in texture, pliant or yielding (MED) neutrytyuus (280) adj., pertaining to the function of nourishing (MED)

nexionam (881) n., regional name for a sty

ny3 (112), adj., nigh, near (MED)

noose (842) = nose

notmygg (792) n., the spice nutmeg (MED)

notys of Indie (244) n., coconuts (MED)

noyous (265) adj., harmful, injurious (MED)

nought (158) nou3t (120) nowght (145) adv., variants of not

nucys Indie (691) nucys Indicem (410) n., coconuts (MED)

o (553) indefinite article (MED)

obtalmie (66) n., ophthalmia, an inflamation of the conjunctiva of the eye (MED)

obticus (16) adj., optic

obtik (88) adj., optic

oynement (392) onement (464) onyment (905) n., ointment, medical salve (MED)

olibam (691) n., frankincense, an aromatic resin used in various ointments (MED)

olibanum album (815) n., white paste of frankincense and water (MED)

opylacion (787) n., obstruction, blockage (MED)

opylate (303) adj., obstructed, blocked (MED)

opon (195) adj., with adv. wide, stretched out supine (MED)

optici (98) adj., optic, genitive case

os (13) conj., as (MED)

ouerkeuery (518) v., to cover over, spread over completely (MED)

ouerlayd (310) ouerleid (778) adj., covered over (MED)

ouerthwart (172) adj., placed crosswise, transversely (MED)

palsye (710) n., failure of a part of the body to function properly, paralysis (MED)

pannycle (428) panniclus (67) n., one of four types of sanguine disease that may affect the conjunctiva *pannum vitreum* (609) n., a glassy or glass-like membrane; the second phlegmatic illness

papulam (882) n., regional name for a sty

parcely (731) n., the herb parsley (MED)

parow (823) n., peeling of a fruit (MED s.v. parure sense 2)

past (1317) n., paste, dough (MED)

pedecelle (432) n., regional name for the first type of pannicle

peyre (62) v., deteriorate, weaken, decline (MED)

pelett (165) pelatis (169) n., sing. and pl., a spherical object, a pill (MED)

perrowr (901) n., peeling of a fruit; cp. parow (MED)

phisyk (3) n., medical science, practice of medicine (MED)

pyllys (498) n., apple peelings (MED s.v. pil(e n. 2))

pillule (165) n., medicinal pill (MED)

pylowe (927) n., a surgical pad or padded dressing (MED)

pyonie (793) pioniorum (794) n., the plant peony (MED)

plaster (193) playster (197) plastrys (149), n., a poltice or compress to be applied to the affected area (MED)

Poile (1289) n., Apulia, a region in southern Italy

poyntes (1079) n. pl., the corners (of the eyes) (MED s.v. pointe sense 12 (b))

polypodie (408) n., common polypody (MED), oak fern (Hunt)

popee (696) n., the poppy, opium poppy (MED)

power (699) v., pour

practyfe (276) n., practitioners

practik (5) n., practical aspect or application of something (MED)

propre (4) adj., own, self (MED)

propriete (224) See Introduction, p. 41

propurly (59) adv., in a manner pertaining to themselves, personal, private (MED)

pulyal (695) n., the herb pennyroyal or wild thyme (MED)

pullyalys (351) n., here = pills

puluerem (390) n., accusative of puluis, powder

puluis benedictus (390) n., a type of powder for treating ophthalmia *puluis nabatis* (415) n., a type of powder made from sugar and soot, specifically for the third type of pannicle

pupilla (48) n., pupil (of the eye)

pustile (1289) n., regional name for a web or pterygium in the eye

putrefacta (156) adj., rotten, putrefied

quarteron (354) n., one fourth of a measure, in this case of an ounce (MED)

queysy (647) adj., of food, unsettling to the stomach, unsuitable (MED)

quibybus (167) n., peppercorn (MED), cubeba (Hunt)

quyk (516) adj., alive, in this case firy (MED)

quyksyluer (287) n., the metal mercury (MED)

rankyll (596) n., a sore, festering sore (MED)

rasoure (478) rasure (628) n., lit. a razor; here, a scalpel (MED)

rechelesly (1168) adv., without regard to the consequences (MED)

rectina (30) n., the retina, the name of one of the tunics or coverings over the eye

rede sawnders (730) n., a mineral substance, red-coloured natron (MED s.v. saun-de-ver)

reynes (469) n., kidneys (MED)

rere (198) adj., of eggs, soft cooked (MED)

rewe (260) n., the herb rue (MED)

roote (992) v., decay, rot (MED)

rothed (1081) roted (153) n., decay, corruption

rotith (153) v., to rot (3rd sing. pres.), translates *putrefieri* VP1, f. 253

rubarbe (409) n., rhubarb (Hunt)

sade (1317) adj., solid, dense, compact (OED)

saferon (245) n., the herb saffron, crocus (MED)

Salernitanum (241) adj., of or pertaining to Salerno, the medical centre in southern Italy; see Introduction, pp. 4, 9–10

saluatrice (41) adj., the name Benvenutus gives to one of the two tunics he acknowledges *sandalus rubeus* (353) n., the powdered wood of the red sandalwood tree (MED)

sandragon (1342) n., the red juice or resin of the dragon tree (MED); translates *sanguis draconis*, VP1, f. 256v

saphyr (753) n., the precious stone sapphire (MED)

Sarazyns (155) n., Arabs or muslims (MED)

sarcacollum album (378) n., a gum exuded by one of several Persian trees (MED); wild briony, wild nep, wild vine, agrimony (Hunt)

Sardonia (650) n., Sardinia, the island to the west of the Italian peninsula

sars (246) sarce (697) v., sift through a sieve (MED)

saunders (813) n., a mineral substance (MED s.v. saun-de-ver)

sause (446) n., sauce, here specifying a degree of fineness: chop the ingredients as finely as you would if making sauce (MED s.v. sauce where this meaning is not noted)

sawge (260) n., the herb sage (MED)

scab (658) skabe (358) n., scabies, specifically an itch on the inner side of the eyelid (MED)

schyt (591) shitt (634) v., shut, close (MED)

scliros (31) n., the name of one of the tunics or coverings over the eye

secundina (31) n., the name of one of the tunics or coverings over the eye

seying (12) n., observation, act of seeing (MED)

seyn (87) v., see (MED)

sensowdid (934) adj., healed; possibly an error for consowded, q.v.

sentence (2) n., opinion, way of thinking (MED)

sercle (47) n., circle

sesyn (1156) v., cease

siler mownten (789) n., a herb, siler montanum, sermountain (Hunt)

synew (16) n., here, a nerve (MED s.v. sineu 2)

sytrynne (140) adj., yellowish in colour

skaldyng (873) adj., lit. burnt, scalded; here, afflicted with a redness that resembles a burn

skume (559) n., froth, foam (MED s.v. scome)

smalache (693) smalege (791) n., the herb smallage, wild celery, celery (MED)

soden (103) adj., cooked, seethed, boiled (MED s.v. sethen)

softlye (190) adv., delicately, carefully (MED)

sokyng (343) adj., slow, damped down (?) (MED)

sotill (522) adj., finely ground (MED)

sotyllye (478) adv., intelligently, carefully, skilfully (MED)

sowden (999) v., to heal (MED)

sowthystyl (638) n., the herb sowthistle, our lady's thistle (MED)

sperages (731) n., a herb, perhaps herb robert? (MED); dove's foot, crane's bill (Hunt)

spice (101) spices (124) n., species (MED)

spygnarde (409) spynarde (692) n., a herb, perhaps Valeriana officinalis (MED); spikenard, galingale (Hunt)

stampe (445) v., to pound, crush, mash (an ingredient) (MED)

step (912) stepe (906) n., the scar left by an injury or infection (MED)

stert (806) v., to burst out of the proper place (MED)

stew (261) n., a bathhouse (MED)

stoke (173) n., lit. a block of wood; here, a bench (MED); translates *scamnum* VP3, f. 98

stoke fysshe (1389) n., a fish dried in the air without salt (MED)

stonye (516) adj., made of stone (MED)

strenus (1001) n., the germinal vesicle in the yolk of an egg (MED s.v. stren)

subtilizen (911) v., to cause a thing to become thinner or less dense (MED s.v. sotilen and subtiliaten)

succum liqueritiae (816) n., juice of liquorice (Hunt).

suger captyu (1255) n., translates *zuccerum captiuum* VP1, f. 255v

swageth (536) n., relieves pain (MED)

swevyng (1072) n., sexual intercourse (MED)

swynge (558) v., to beat, whip, as of eggs (MED)

temper (341) v., to mingle, mix (OED)

temperate (111) adj., tempered, modified (OED)

thyrl (179) v., to pierce (OED)

thow (295) conj., though

tonicle (46) tunicle (29) n., the tunic or coat that covers the eye (OED)

torturam tenebrosam (387) n., Benvenutus's name for ophthalmia

towe (passim) though, in the phrase "as towe"

tremelyng (287) adj., trembling (OED)

turbite (166) n., turpath, a cathartic drug prepared from the root of the East Indian jalap; also the plant itself or its root (OED); cp. Hunt s.v. tora

Tuscia (619) n., Tuscany, a region of central Italy

tutie (340) tutie of Alexander (1274) n., a crude or impure oxide of zinc (OED)

twych (847) twycchys (477) n., in the sing., poss. a hook, poss. tweezers; pl. tweezers (OED); translates *uncino* VP1, f. 249; *uncinum argenti* VP1, f. 252

vele (128) adv., well

vertu youen of god (1186) n., another name for the salve *virtus a deo data*

vexen (783) v., to wax, become

vyolence (1256) n., of medicines, strength, potency (OED)

virtus a deo data (999) n., name of a salve invented by Benvenutus

uitacelle (732) n., properly vitiscella; the herb red and white briony (Hunt)

vitreus (97) uitrius (35) adj., the name of one of the three liquids or humours in the eye

vngle (848) vngyll (841) n., fr L *vngula*, a (finger)nail, a pterygium or tumour on the conjunctiva of the eye (OED)

vnguentum alabastrum (914) n., an ointment prescribed by Benvenutus

vnguentum subtile (907) n., an ointment prescribed by Benvenutus

vngula (835) n., a (finger)nail; i.e., a pterygium or tumour on the conjunctiva of the eye (OED)

vnneth (747) adv., scarcely, barely (OED)

voydyth (954) v., discharges, expels (matter) from an infection (OED s.v. void, sense 7 by analogy to an unnatural vent or orifice)

urtice ultra marine (790) n., the sea nettle (?) (OED). VP1, f. 251v urtice
    trans marine uel ciciliane

vtter (943) adj., outer

vuea (31) n., the name of one of the tunics or coverings over the eye

wacche (801) n., wakefulness, vigil (OED)

walworte (664) n., the herb dwarfelder, ground elder (OED); Danewort
    (Hunt)

wareþorwe (45) conj., wherethrough, through which

warly (629) adv., carefully, prudently (OED)

watche (139) n., wakefulness, vigil (OED)

webbys (67) n. pl., thin, white film or opacity growing over the eye;
    perhaps a pterygium or ungula (OED)

well (14) n., translation of *fonte*, found in some manuscripts instead of
    fronte, to describe the location of the eyes

weryly (961) adv., warely, carefully, prudently (OED)

wete (766) v., to know

wherthrugh (424) conj., wherethrough, through which

whitnesse (72) n., whiteness

wyde opon (195) adj., stretched out flat on the back, supine (OED)

wykkyd (132) adj., harmful, dangerous (OED)

wyse (208) n., way, manner, fashion (OED)

withtempere (543) v., a nonce word meaning to mix or mingle with;
    translates *contemperat* (VP1, f. 249v), taking its prefix literally

wytsayff (1384) v., vouchesafe, confer, bestow (OED)

wodenes (548) n., violence, fierceness, ferocity (OED)

wonde (925) n., = wound

wormewode (1033) n., the herb artemisia absinthium (OED)

worschype (483) n., honour, renown (OED)

wryth (180) v., to twist back and forth in the manner of a drill (OED)

wulgalpus (956) n., a nonce word (?), perhaps a misreading of *muru et*
    vulgariter cersu (VP1, f. 253), taking *vulgariter* for a noun?

yere (1196) = ear [e.g., of wheat or other grain]